The Storm Unseen

The Storm Unseen

A Memoir of Life with Lupus

LILLIAN MAKLE FORBES

Xulon Press

Xulon Press
2301 Lucien Way #415
Maitland, FL 32751
407.339.4217
www.xulonpress.com

Unless otherwise indicated, Scripture quotations taken from the HOLY
BIBLE, New International Version (NIV). Copyright © 1973, 1978,
1984, 2011 by Biblica, Inc.™. Used by permission. All rights reserved.

Printed in the United States of America.

Edited by Xulon Press.

ISBN-13: 9781545640982

Dedicated to these special people in my life.

James H. Forbes, Jr. (My wonderful husband)
Daryl (Boo) Hall (nephew)
Lillian E. Makle (mother)
Michelle R. Forbes (daughter)
Sheree N. Forbes (daughter)
Pastor Sandra E. Smith (sister)
Jean Harding (babysitter)

TABLE OF CONTENTS

ACKNOWLEDGMENTS

My nephew Daryl "Boo" Hall gave me the ultimate Gift of life and a sacrifice of a kidney. After my battle with lupus for twelve years I needed a kidney transplant. Words can never express my gratitude towards him for what he did for me. I love Boo with all of my heart.

I thank my husband, a strong man of God, who stood right by my side and he still stands with me today treating me as his queen.

I thank God for my sweet, sweet mother whose heart ached for me. She was strong for me when I could not be strong for myself.

I thank God for my sister, Pastor Sandra Smith, who never left my side and encouraged me through every dark and deep valley. I also thank God for the pastors of several local churches who prayed for me.

I thank God for my brothers and sisters who were there for me to encourage me. There is nothing greater than having a family who believes in prayer and knows the power of prayer.

I thank God for my babysitter Ms. Jean Harding who took care of me and my children the entire time I was ill. I love her and owe her so much.

I thank God for my in-laws who were there for support and encouragement. I also thank God for my friends who encouraged me along the way. Last but not least, I thank the doctors and nurses of Georgetown University Hospital, Johns Hopkins Hospital, and Fresenius Dialysis Center of Waldorf, Maryland, for their professionalism, compassion, support, and encouragement.

Give thanks to the Lord, for he is good, his love endures forever.
(First Chronicles 16:34)

INTRODUCTION

My obstetrician told me on May 27, 1994, while in my eighth
month of pregnancy, that I might have a chronic disease
called lupus. It was a devastating time for me in a way that I would
never think would be possible. This was a chronic disease that I
knew nothing about. Likewise, it was an emotional time because
I feared the unknown of what any type of chronic disease could
do. I remember reading stories about how people can die from
lupus, and I did not want that to happen to me. All I could do was
sit in the chair, frozen in my body and my mind, trying to figure
out if this was a dream or reality while I stared out the window
watching and counting the cars going up and down the highway. It
was like having an out-of-body experience. This was shocking to
me because I thought I was always healthy for the most part, but
I had no idea that I lived with a chronic disease that could take
my life. My and my husband's plans were to start thinking about
adding to our family, not going into the doctor's office and hearing
of some chronic disease that we knew nothing about. It just made
us feel that we should forget about all of our plans and forget about
ever being happy again.

I can only remember the doctors telling me that I had systemic
lupus erythematous ("lupus"). Later, I developed cutaneous (discoid) lupus. This form of lupus is limited to the skin. It can cause
many types of rashes and lesions or sores in the mouth. The rashes

are raised, scaly, and red and itch from time to time. It is called discoid lupus because the rash is shaped like discs, or circles. The systemic lupus erythematous is the most common form of lupus. It can be mild or severe. Unlike the discoid lupus, this form of lupus attacks major organ systems in the body. Some of the serious complications are inflammation of the kidneys (lupus nephritis), increase in blood pressure in the lungs (pulmonary hypertension), or inflammation of the brain's blood vessels. The doctors told me there is no cure for this chronic disease, but medicines would help keep it under control as long as I took them properly.

Chapter 1

"WHAT IS THIS, LUPUS?" /
THE FACTS

In case you don't know what lupus is, lupus is a chronic autoimmune disease that can damage any part of the body, whether the skin, joints, or organs. The word *chronic* pertaining to lupus means the signs and symptoms of the disease persist longer than six weeks and often for years. Doctors say there is no known cure, but only different courses of treatment.

I was given facts and information about the disease by my rheumatologist, my nephrologists, at Johns Hopkins University in Baltimore, Maryland and by the Lupus Foundation of America, of which I am a member in the Washington DC chapter. *(Lahita, 1994)* They sent me different brochures on what I needed to know about the disease, and how it might affect my body and my life because it affects everyone differently. They also sent a special brochure on African Americans and lupus because it is known to be more common in African Americans.

Lupus can change the quality of your life when it affects your autoimmune system. *(ibid.)*

Your antibodies are attacking your own body, and it is hard for your body to fight because it cannot tell the healthy body tissues from the foreign invaders that can attack your body, like bacteria, viruses, flu, and germs. These are the things that go wrong with your immune system, which causes extreme pain and inflammation in various parts of your body. People with lupus tend to have flare-ups where the disease gets worse, and the body begins to shut down in certain areas. My body had too many flare-ups. I was in and out of the hospital often.

Lupus affected me in more ways than one. I had the cutaneous (discoid) lupus, which affects the skin. It usually presents as a red rash that appears on the skin, such as the neck, face, and scalp. The rash will sometimes have pus in it.

The rash spreads across the forehead, along the bridge of the nose, and covers the cheeks. It is usually called "the butterfly rash" because of its wing shape on the face. I also developed black lesions over my face, arms, legs, and back that have left permanent scars and lesions on my body. I call them my "battle scars" for the victory that I did not see ahead of me.

Systemic lupus erythematous is the other type of lupus that I had. It is more serious because it affects not only the skin, but other parts of the body such as joints, kidneys, heart, lungs, brain, and the blood. I incurred all of the symptoms from this horrible disease. I had the rashes and the lesions, scaly dry skin, sores in my nose and mouth, and joint pain and swelling, and I felt fatigued all the time. I lost almost all of my hair, with just enough to cover the scalp. It was difficult for me to eat because the sores in my mouth were so painful. Even with all my hair gone, I refused to buy a wig to cover my hair loss. I felt emptiness and self-pity because there was a time when the Lord had blessed me with a beautiful head of flowing, long healthy hair that hung down my back, and that was how everyone knew me. All of my life I would get so many compliments on my hair, so losing it was traumatizing. I knew hair does not make a person who they are, but it shows a sign of identity for that person. I thought I was so ugly because of the facial changes, scars, and hair loss. I felt like I had truly lost my sense of identity and what I looked like. It left me with low self-esteem, and I did not want anyone to see me. Hair is a blessing from God and 1 Corinthians 11:15 says, "but that if a woman has long hair, it is her glory, for long hair is given to her as a covering," and we as women also see hair as a form of attractiveness. When we lose it all, it takes us to a place of feeling unattractive and having little self-worth.

I felt like purchasing a wig would be a cover-up for all that I had been through already. I felt like something—or someone—had stolen my identity when I was diagnosed with lupus. Everything about who I was and what I looked like for so long disappeared from my life. I did not want people to see the "real me" and what I had become at this time in my life. This was a defense mechanism for me, as I refused to accept my new reality.

It was hard for me to go outside and be stared at because of how I looked, on top of having no hair. I was not ready to handle my emotional state along with what people could be thinking about me. Still, I had to go outside in order to go back and forth to the doctor. So, I would tie my head up with a scarf, which helped, but that did not help with the look of my face and my skin. I felt like this was how I would look for the rest of my life—if I had a rest of my life—so I might as well accept who and what I was going to look like regardless, so a wig was not an option I wanted to take. If I bought a wig, I would have been in more denial and not able to face this part of reality in my life.

I remember trying all different types of makeup to hide my facial lesions and discoloration, but no matter what makeup it was or how expensive, the lesions and the rash always showed through. I even went to a dermatologist for a cream or medicine for my face. I was given something to diminish the lesions, but I felt so ugly because people would stare at me. The way I looked when I saw myself in the mirror was the way I felt other people saw me, and that was hard for me to accept.

The ninety-five milligrams of prednisone gave such an ugly look to my face and to my body. Each day, I walked past the mirror, and I tried not to look at myself because all I saw was this ugly person because the high dose of prednisone caused so many different and unusual changes to my body. I felt like my body went through a metamorphosis in many different stages.

It started with a large round "moon face." A high dose of prednisone causes your face to become large and round, like the shape of a full moon. The medical term is Cushing's syndrome in which extra fat builds up around the sides of your face. *(Chang-Miller, 2011)* As if that was not enough, I had to look at my abdomen that would never go down; my stomach had such a weird shape to it after the baby. It was a large hump shape that appeared from under my chest cavity to the lower part of my stomach. My stomach had marks on both sides that pointed directly up to my navel area. In reality, they looked like a road map to me. They were stretch marks, but they turned extremely red and began to spread around the bottom of my stomach. The doctor called it abdominal striate (stripes), and she explained this happens when you are on an extremely high dose of prednisone. I still looked as though I was pregnant, but the shape of my stomach was a long awkward egg shape that protruded outward from my body.

There was also a large hump in the back of neck, which, according to the medical terminology, is called the "buffalo hump" in which fat deposits build up because of too much prednisone in the system. My clothes would sit up on the back of my neck because of how noticeable the buffalo hump was. I also began to notice I was starting to grow fine facial hair along the sides of my face by my ears, which made it look like I had sideburns. My doctor called this hirsutism, which is excessive growth of body hair. *Lloyd, William C.,III, 2016), https://www.healthgrades.com* All of these symptoms were side effects from this one powerful drug. It all made me look and feel so deformed. My eyes were constantly bloodshot both from the lupus and the medicines.

One day I stood in the mirror and told myself that I hated the way I looked and hated my life that I lived. I pulled at the strands of my hair, and as I cried, I could hear the Lord's voice so plain in my ear saying to me softly and peacefully, "The Lord gives and the Lord taketh away."

I did not want to hear that because it did not make me feel any better about myself. I became numb toward life and myself.

Each time I was exposed to the sun, I felt sick and drained. I had frequent memory loss, protein in my urine, a low red and white blood cell count, and the most devastating of all, renal failure.

It was heartbreaking and overwhelming to receive this type of news when I was eight months pregnant. I had no idea if I, or the baby, would live, or what my life would be like.

I knew in my heart that I loved God, and in my mind I knew that God loved me. The traumatizing news that I received of having this chronic disease was very hard for me to accept.

No matter how afraid or mad I was, I had to trust Almighty God to heal me and bring me through.

This is my story of my catastrophic illness and how it has changed my life forever.

Come and hear, all you who fear God; let me tell you what he has done
I cried out to him with my mouth; his praise was on my tongue.
If I had cherished sin in my heart, the Lord would not have listened;
but God has surely listened and has heard my prayer.
Praise be to God,
who has not rejected my prayer or withheld his love from me!
(Psalm 66:16-20)

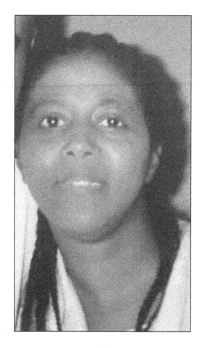

Chapter 2

MY PREGNANCY AND LUPUS

I lay upstairs in my bed on a hot summer morning in August; I rocked back and forth in the fetal position. I didn't care whether I lived or died. I tried to understand what storm I had just walked into.

It all began for me when I was admitted to Georgetown University Hospital on May 28, 1994. I was there for a month, when I was only supposed to go there to give birth to a baby. During the month I was in the hospital, the day of June 30, 1994, loomed closer and closer—the day I was scheduled to go home with my newborn baby girl. I dreaded it.

I had given birth to this darling angel sent from God named Sheree whom I was too sick to care for. I also had an eight-year-old daughter waiting to see her new baby sister and me, and yet, I was too sick to be a mother to either of them. I was sick to the point of death.

Yet, I knew I had to come home and face the unknown of my life. After giving birth to this breathtaking baby girl, the only thought that ran through my mind was how I was going to take care of this child, someone so small and so precious.

After I laid eyes on her, I said to myself, *oh how beautiful she is to me*. She had such smooth chocolate brown skin and straight black hair. She had a head full of it. She was the most adorable baby in the world to me.

I didn't want to go home because I knew if I stayed in the hospital, the doctors would take good care of me. I was on a regimen of thirteen medications a day, including ninety-five milligrams of prednisone, which is a synthetic corticosteroid that acts as an anti-inflammatory medication to treat diseases that affect the immune system. I was on insulin because I had to check my blood sugar three or four times a day, not because I was a diabetic, but because of all the high doses of medications that caused my blood sugar to spike from 150 to 350 from time to time.

I knew nothing about any of the medications or how to take them. Still, I felt as long as I could stay in the hospital, the doctors were familiar with all of my medicines and how I should be taking them.

I was afraid that if I came home, I would surely die because I had no awareness to realize how sick I truly was. I felt safe being in the hospital. I knew the nurses would be able to care for my baby when I could not.

There were many times the nurses would bring my baby to me, and I would tell them to take her away because I did not want her knowing I could not care for her. I felt no love and compassion for this adorable baby that a mother should feel after giving birth. I was sad and depressed that I had this new little life, but without the joy or excitement in my heart to even hold her. I could only think about myself and what would happen to me.

Finally, on the morning of June 28, the doctors and a nurse came into my room with smiles on their faces to tell me that they had wonderful news.

I wanted them to tell me, "The lupus is gone and your body has returned back to normal."

I wanted them to tell me, "Mrs. Forbes, you will not have to take all of these medications anymore."

Instead, they came to tell me that they felt like I was able to go home and they would go over all of my medications with me. I did not want to hear that. They stood in front of me with a list and instructions of all my medications and how I was supposed to take them. While they spoke to my husband and me, I found myself slowly detaching from the conversation.

They told me that I would be able to rest more and that they would stay in close communication with me to make sure I made progress with the medicines and my baby.

"Please let me stay longer," I begged them. "I'm not ready to go home; I'm not prepared mentally, physically, or emotionally to take care of this baby. Bringing this baby home with me is too much to bear. Can't you see with all of the medications I'm taking, I cannot take care of myself and I cannot take care of this child?"

While looking at them with tears rolling down my face, I pleaded with the nurse, "Just talk to my obstetrician because I just can't do this."

Then the nurse looked at me with concern and confidence and said, "Mrs. Forbes, you will be okay, and you'll have someone there to help you."

Even though she tried to convince me I would not be alone once I was home, I still did not want to go.

As the day drew closer for me to be released from the hospital, the nurses came in my room, opened the curtains, and said, "Let some sunshine in! We're bringing in your bundle of joy."

They brought the baby into my room so I could become familiar with having a newborn. They watched while I held her to make sure I held her correctly. It was so hard for me to adjust to being a mother after all this time, and the scariest part was having to take care of this child knowing I was not physically and mentally capable, though the doctors thought differently. It would be hard for me to even hold this baby because I had no emotions or love in me to show her. I had to force myself to hold her in my arms and try to show her some affection.

I remember the ride home felt like such a long way. I felt like we rode for hours and hours in my mind while the hot sun beat down on the window, even though the trip took only one hour. I remember crying the entire way home because I had not been outside the hospital for nearly a month. All I knew for a month was doctors and nurses bringing me medication every day while I lay in that hospital bed, counting the flowers on the wallpaper—tiny pink tulips on a beige background with small green leaves on each side. I know there must have been at least a one hundred of them on that wall because I would program my mind to stare and count them, hoping when I was done counting, everything would be over.

I secretly wished we would never get home, or that my family would somehow get there without me. Having this new addition to our family was supposed to be a happy time for my husband and me. We were so excited about expanding our family like we had dreamed. Yet, things did not turn out the way we had imagined, and dreams don't always come true.

In my mind, our dream had turned into a nightmare that I did not want to wake up to and a reality that I could not face. If I could have sent my husband and baby home without me, it would have been easier for me to suffer in silence, knowing I would not be a burden to my family.

I felt like they deserved a life of happiness as a family, not having to carry the burden of taking care of an ill woman—someone who was supposed to be a mother and wife. I wanted him to leave me in the hospital as a long-term patient or put me somewhere until I got better. That way, I could be the mother and wife I was supposed to be when I was able and healthy. This, however, is not how it was supposed to be.

I continued looking out the window as we took the endless drive home. Thoughts went through my mind as we drove toward home. Thoughts of agony, fear, and pain hit me harder the closer we got to home. The thoughts smothered my mind. The closer we got, the more fearful I became. I wanted to yell to my husband, "Stop the car! Turn around. Take me back to the hospital!"

Yet, I knew I couldn't. Just the thought of being responsible for a little helpless life terrified me because I too was helpless to even care for myself.

Who would take care of me? Who would make sure I took all of those medications correctly and when I needed them? When the baby needed feeding or changing, who would do that? Who would give this newborn the attention she needs? I needed someone to help me every minute of the day.

Who would check my blood pressure? Who would check my blood sugar and give me my insulin when I needed to take it? The doctors and nurses were at the hospital, and they did it all for me. I felt safe in that hospital. I felt I had a chance to live, not a chance to die.

My heart felt numb, like there was no love in it anymore, not even for this baby girl that I was supposed to love, bond with, and mother.

All I could think about was what had happened to me. I lived in my worst nightmare, and I never was able to wake up. And I wanted stay in that state until I died. I just had a baby, and my body showed all of the scars and stretch marks after a caesarian birth, but I had no baby to bond with. I did not have my other daughter to hold and tell her everything was going to be okay. All I had was a dresser full of thirty medications lined up for me to take, a notebook and tablet with all the times my husband was supposed to give me the medication, and a baby's nursery decorated so perfectly with baby pictures, carousels hanging from the crib that was full of baby gifts, and a rocking chair that I was supposed to be in, bonding with Sheree.

There was no baby, and there was no Michelle, my eight-year-old daughter. My dear neighbor was the babysitter for Michelle, and like a grandmother, she offered to take my baby and let her stay with her while I tried to get well. My mother took Michelle to stay with her.

There was this newborn baby I brought with me and my eight-year-daughter Michelle waiting for me, and then there was my mind that I felt like I had slowly lost. I wanted to be the normal mother who goes into the hospital to give birth to her child and comes home. If only this was a dream, but it wasn't. It was a reality that I did not want to face.

I had no mental and physical ability to do or feel anything, except wishing I was dead. Just the awful thoughts of trying to adapt to a major life change, along with so many medical issues all at one time, was enough to make me feel like I had truly lost my mind. My house was not the house I left. This was not the loving family I left. This was a different life that I knew nothing about or how to live. I remember the doctors telling my husband that they would make arrangements for him to have an in-house nurse to come out twice a week to check my vitals, to check the protein in my urine, and to also make sure I had adapted to my new life because of all the medications and possible side effects they could have. She would come on Tuesdays and Thursday to talk with me and to examine me to make sure I did everything on a regular basis. I remember her saying, "Mrs. Forbes, I know it's hard, but you have a beautiful baby and a loving husband. It is going to be okay."

That did not matter to me because she could not feel the pain and hurt that I felt. No matter how encouraging kind words can sound, when your heart is torn apart, it will only take the love and grace of God to repair it.

This was an overload to my brain and my body, and I couldn't deal with any of it. No matter how much I wished things would be different, they stayed the same. Each day, the depression sank deeper and deeper; the pain was a gut-wrenching pain in my heart and stomach that would never go away. I felt like I was not living in reality anymore. It's like walking and slowly feeling your feet disappearing from under you, and before you realize it, you have fallen. I know I had a family, and I know I gave birth, but I would ask, *God, what has happened to my life?*

The pain in my stomach hurt so bad because of all the medications, and cesarean birth and all of the staples, and excessive swelling from the medications, but the pain in my heart was the worst. I asked myself over and over, *where is the family I thought I had made? The one I thought I was coming home to?* I cried for my life to be normal every day, but the "normal" I once knew felt so far away.

In my bedroom, which I looked at as a prison, were lavender walls trimmed in white, gorgeous soft purple curtains hung from the windows, and bright pictures on the walls. Once I was home from the hospital, I had to be in my bed with my feet propped on four large pillows because of the tremendous swelling in my legs and ankles. I had no contact with anyone except for a few phone calls, and every now and then, my neighbor would come by and check on me. She would bring my baby girl over twice a week just so I could look at her. And that broke my heart. She was my baby, and I should have had her with me.

What I saw in my mind was this prison that I was trapped in, never having a "normal" life again. I had to talk to myself and try to convince myself that things would get better and that this would not last forever. Still, every day I woke up with the same feelings in the same dark place. Looking around my bedroom, I remembered how excited I was when we painted the walls. I told my husband, "This is what a royal bedroom looks like."

I could not fathom that what I once thought was so beautiful was such a horrible place to be in.

I wanted the curtains drawn, but that still did not stop the sun from shining through. I wanted to drown myself in the darkness of the room because the self-pity was a comfortable place for me. The darkness in my room was a satisfying place for me because I felt so dark in my mind. In that place, I felt a source of contentment.

No matter how dark my situation was in my life, in my mind I would tell myself over and over, *God is here, and He is protecting me and keeping me.* I believed in the Lord all of my life and as I grew older, I grew closer to God, but at this time in my life, I felt like He was nowhere to be found. I felt abandoned by Him. Yet, I knew deep in my heart He already knew what I would go through and what I would face in this life. He still kept the sun shining through those dark curtains to remind me of what He says in His Word. I would repeat this verse every day to myself from Deuteronomy 31:8: "The Lord said He is the one who goes before you, He will be with you," and He goes on to say, "I will never leave you nor forsake you."

He tried to reach me through my pain, but I failed to see He took all of my pain, hurt, sickness, and sins to the cross with Him. Though I went through hell in the flesh, He had already taken care of it for me. I saw it as the sunshine being the Holy Spirit, reminding me that the Son Jesus Christ was with me the whole time. I believed I was the apple of God's eye and that is how He sees me and that is how much He loves me. Yet, I didn't want to get out of bed. I did not want to wash my body, comb what little hair I had left, or even eat. I did not want to do anything but think about how my life could have been with a wonderful husband and children. My life before all of this felt like a fairy tale where the princess marries the prince who treated her like his wonderful jewel.

Still, no matter how I tried to keep the curtains drawn and light out, my husband would say, "Let some sun shine in here; it will make you feel better."

But I still wanted them drawn. I believe that the sun was Almighty God trying to tell me, "I will not and I have not left you."

At this time God was the last person that I wanted to hear from, no matter how much He kept the sun shining in that dark place.

My heart and mind did not care about the sunshine while I lay in my bed, crying tears that I wished no one could see or hear. I knew my family loved me, but they faced not only my health, but also the health of my father. They were afraid they would lose me and my dad, who was diagnosed with terminal cancer at the same time I was diagnosed with lupus. I felt like it was all too much for them to handle and process at one time. I had a chronic illness that none of us knew anything about but had only heard from others how people pass away from this disease. As my father lay so sick, I felt like I was the last thing they should worry about.

I believed God did not care about what was happening to me because if He did, why had He allowed this terrible disease to enter my body and change my life forever? I was mad at God, and I couldn't understand, so I had to keep asking God, "Why, why are you doing this to me?"

I told myself all day as I cried out to Him, "Other people have sinned. I did not murder anyone. I did not commit a big crime, so why are you doing this to me? God, I have tried to live right, live according to your Holy Word, so what have I done to make you do this to me? Why? Why don't you love me anymore, God? Why are you punishing me this way?"

My human nature wanted me to believe this should not have happened to me. I felt like I had done all the right things, so I did not deserve this devastating storm I was in. I felt like God didn't see the good I had done, and he only wanted to punish me along with others who did bad. My mind was not able to snap out of those thoughts. I was not spiritually equipped to handle the battles when they came because they came too fast. We as humans think nothing traumatic will happen to us if we are living right. Still, I had to learn that as well as we try to live by the Word of God, we are not exempt from trials and tribulations, and it is hard for us to trust God will do what He says He will do.

We all struggle because the world pulls at our flesh. Yet, it is all in how you handle the battle. Matthew 5:45 states that God causes the rain to fall on both the just and the unjust.

I felt like I was struggling to breathe as someone held me underwater and made me hold my breath, knowing I cannot swim. Every time I inhaled felt like labor pains. Everywhere I turned in my bedroom and in my home, there was no fresh air, only a suffocating feeling. My life felt void of all oxygen.

I could remember the smell of the fresh air in my mind and see the summer flowers in the garden when I would get out of bed and go to the window. Though the carpet was soft on my feet, they were so swollen and tight that it hurt to put any pressure on them by standing. I did not want to get up and have to look across the hall at my baby's room. It was a daily reminder that my life as I knew it was gone.

My life felt cold, lonely, forlorn, and empty. I knew my family loved me, but because they had their own lives, I could not expect them to be there for me every day. I knew that was not possible because my mother needed my other siblings to be her support and strength while my father was terminally ill.

Though my mother was a strong Christian woman who loved the Lord, the news of both of our illnesses devastated her and the rest of my family.

All I could feel was I needed my mother. As selfish as it sounds, I wanted her with me. My family would call to check on me and check with my husband to see what they could do to help, but I needed and wanted my mom there because I was scared, and I could not do this without her, but my father needed her also. My husband did so much for me, and my neighbor would cook my meals three times a day. Even though she did her best, along with my husband, I still felt alone. My heart felt crushed, and I didn't care if I ever had another heartbeat again. We were a close-knit family, but I could not accept that they could not come to see about me as much as I wanted them to because of my dad's illness and the need to be there for my mom.

Yes, I would get upset with them, and I would take my anger out on my husband and ask him, "How come they can't come and see about me? Why can't they cry with me and see the pain and hurt I feel?"

They left me to handle this by myself. I wanted them to share in my pain. Yet, they were not there with me. I was afraid, and I needed them. My father passed away on August 28, 1995, after being diagnosed with lung cancer in November of 1993. That was a terrible time for my family. I could not comprehend my father had died because my mind was still not there. It took me a few years to process that my father had passed.

After my appointment at Johns Hopkins one evening, my husband and decided it would be best if we took Michelle to my mother's house so she could care for her. We knew Michelle would be safe with her grandmother to love her and try to help her to understand what her mommy was going through at that time.

We waited for Michelle to come home from school, and we sat her down to explain to her what we needed to do for our family. After we talked, she and I went into her bedroom, and we began to pack her clothes and some of her favorite books and toys, and we planned on taking her bike, which she loved to ride. I tried to make the drive to my mom's as fun as possible; we even stopped for ice cream along the way. I reminded her of how she would be playing with her cousins and how she would have a good time with her grandmother until I was able to come back to get her.

As I stood in my mother's yard, I felt hopeless; I saw pain and disappointment in my baby girl's eyes. It was as though she felt like I didn't love her or want her.

Michelle looked up at me and said, "Mommy, I don't want to stay. Please let me come back home with you, please."

Because I had never been without my children, I felt as though I had abandoned her, even though she was with my family. My heart felt as though it was being ripped apart because I knew my baby girl did not understand. This was too much for me to handle. I never wanted to think I had to turn my child away at such a young age when she needed me the most. She kept saying, "Mommy, I want to go home with you. I won't bother you. I will stay in my room. I can watch TV while you rest." My heart was even more broken because she cried and said, "Mommy I can take care of myself. I can fix my own cereal."

All I could say was, "Michelle, you know how much Mommy loves you, but I can't take care of you right now because I am too sick. Please try to understand."

I kept trying my best to explain to her how sick I was, but that did not make the pain any easier for any of us, especially my little girl.

I knew I could not do any of the things we did together anymore because I was in no condition physically and mentally to take care of her, and I know she could not take care of me. I wanted her with me, but I also did not want her with me because she saw all I had to deal with, and I saw how it affected her.

Michelle got off the bike and ran to me, clinging for dear life; she clutched me so hard I felt like we both would fall. Finally, my mom gently pulled her away from me and said, "Michelle, it is going to be okay; your mommy will be back to get you soon."

My mother was upset and heartbroken too, but she knew she had to be strong for Michelle while also dealing with my dad's illness.

As we walked to the car, I could not hold back my tears. My husband tried his best to be strong for the both of us. As I got into the car, I could not stand to look back because I did not want to see and feel the pain that I left in my little girl's heart that day. That broke my heart even more, and I still feel guilt for not being able to keep my daughter with me. Yet, there I was, sick to the point of wishing to die, having to tell her she cannot come home with me. That is something I never want to experience in this life again.

Even though I had a wonderful family, in my mind, no one understood what I went through or how I felt. I felt so much sadness and loneliness for sending my children away to different people while trying to cope with this devastating, chronic illness.

Trust in the Lord with all your heart and lean not on your own understanding;
In all your ways submit to him, and he will make your paths straight.
(Proverbs 3:5-6)

Chapter 3

THE STORM UNSEEN

Sometimes, in the mornings, the rain beat against the window of my bedroom. This constant battering made me feel like the world had closed in on me. *What happened to my life; what happened to me?*

Here I was, this young lady who had had a wonderful life. I felt I was attractive and healthy, I had a great husband, and we were starting a family. I worked as a file clerk in the records section of the Department of Justice, which is considered one of the most prestigious government agencies in the world. We would spend our Sundays in church as a family, and we did our best to read the Word of God. We attended Bible study and enjoyed family time with my brothers and sisters. I felt like the Lord had blessed us abundantly to accomplish all of the things our hearts had desired, because we were so happy.

I was happily married and felt as though God had sent me my soul mate and my best friend. We had our fair share of disagreements like most couples, but we felt happiness every day.

I was the fifth out of ten children: six girls and four boys. My siblings and I were close in age. We grew up on a tobacco farm in a small town called Brandywine, Maryland. My father worked as a laborer with the federal government, and he also worked on his tobacco farm while my mother sometimes did domestic work, such as cleaning houses for the elderly. Though my sisters always called me my dad's "favorite" and felt he spoiled me, I saw things differently.

On the hot summer days when we had to go into the tobacco field to pull grass, I didn't have to go because of my nosebleeds. As a child, I always remembered having a lot of nosebleeds and kidney infections. There were different times when I would have to stay in the hospital for kidney infections that lasted two or three days. I never thought anything would ever evolve from having so many nosebleeds and infections. I would often ask myself why I had to be the one who had some kind of defect, something as stupid as nosebleeds. Two of my brothers would also have nosebleeds, but theirs never appeared to be as severe as mine.

I remember when my mother took me to the doctor for my nosebleeds, and they told her I had anemia, which caused my nose-bleeds. My grandmother and my aunt had a remedy for the nose bleeds. They told my parents to sit me in a chair with my head tilted slightly back, and they would put an icepack in my back, and sometimes they would take a cold butter knife and lay it in my back. I never understood it, but it worked at the time. The bleed-ings continued through my years as a child, so the doctor sug-gested they perform a cauterization to my nose. The doctor would go in my nostrils and seal off the blood vessels so that scar tissue would build up to prevent bleeding. They also told her that they thought I might have a trait of sickle cell blood disorder because of my white blood cell count, which was low at the time, and the white cell count means that the body can be susceptible to illness or infection, which can spiral into a serious health threat that can cause autoimmune diseases.

Yet, as time went on and I grew older, the nosebleeds and the kidney infections begin to stop. I was healthy and could begin to pursue a life and a career. I saw an ad for a job with the Department of Justice in Washington, DC. I thought if I could work there, I could advance in an exciting career. Back in those days, it was important to work for the government because it was a steady, safe job.

I began working as a file clerk in the Records Management Division for the Department of Justice on April 17, 1978. As time went on, I applied for other jobs and I was blessed to receive a promotion as a voucher clerk in the payroll division. I was only nineteen years old, and I felt like I was on top of the world. I still lived at home with my parents, and I had no desire to move out.

It was at my job where I met my wonderful husband, and he became the love of my life. We were married on September 17, 1983, at a St. Michael's Catholic Church in Brandywine, Maryland. We were both young when we got married—I was twenty-four, and James was twenty-six—but we both knew we were in love with each other and that was what we wanted to do. After three years of marriage, we both decided we were ready to start our family. We felt we were more mature and somewhat financially ready to start adding to our family.

When I found out I was pregnant with my first child, my doctor noticed some strange things going on with my blood. My white blood cell would fluctuate from low to high some months, and then my red blood cell count would be high, so they were concerned because they would also see small amounts of protein in the urine, but not anything for them to see a reason to be alarmed. To be cautious, my obstetrician sent me to a hematologist to have my blood checked. He said it would not stay stable. As time went on, I continued my obstetrician appointments, and my doctor decided to put me on extra vitamins and insisted I take it easy until I deliver. They never could find out why my white blood cell count was not normal, so he said I was probably anemic from the pregnancy.

On August 26, 1986, I gave birth to Michelle Renee Forbes. She became the love of our life; we enjoyed being parents, and of course, since she was our first child, we made it a point to spoil her. We had such a loving family, and we enjoyed life to its fullest. However, like many other families, we had our rough moments, but we were a family with a lot of love that went to everyone. Being from such a large family, I knew I wanted to have more than one child.

Take delight in the Lord, and he will give you the desires of your heart.
Commit your way to the Lord; trust in him and he will do this:
He will make your righteous reward shine like the dawn, your vindication like the noonday sun.
(Psalm 37:4-6)

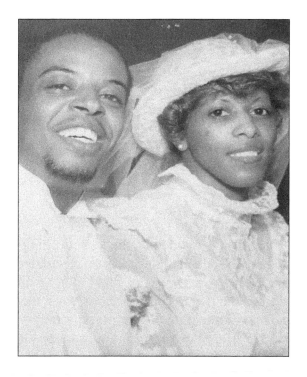

Chapter 4

GOD, WHERE ARE YOU?

W hen I was sick, I would often think about going outside and standing in the rain until the rain would wash me away from the face of the earth. I wanted to die, and I didn't want anyone to save me. I wanted the rain to come, because when the rain comes, it is cold and leaves a feeling of gloom, especially for someone in a bad place in life. Standing in the rain made me feel like I had connected to something unnatural because I would always see a rainbow at the end of a rainy day, especially when there was thunder and lightning. I felt like the rain was all of my human tears falling upon me.

I also wanted the rain to take me to a place of serenity where I would be washed clean from all that had happened to me. If the rain wouldn't cleanse me, then I wanted to stay in it until I disappeared. Still, I wanted to believe because of how I was raised that there was something spiritual about the rainfall.

As a child, I always believed rain was a symbol of cleansing that God brings upon the earth. Rain washes the earth of all its impurities, bringing what is dead back to life. I felt that if I stood in it long enough, He would wash it all away. I felt like He would look at my life and take away the sins that I felt I committed in order to bring this devastating disease upon me. That way, my body and my life would return back to normal and better than it was before. I would be able to open the curtains of my room and let the sunshine come in because I knew God had washed it all away.

I wanted to walk outside and feel a sunny spring day and take in all of God's creation: the beautiful trees, the green grass, and the wind softly blowing. The birds would be flying through the air, constantly giving God praise. That was my fairytale if I went outside to stand in the rain. I felt God would it make all beautiful like a warm and sunny spring day. I looked for that rainbow because it is one of His promises that He gave Noah. God said in Genesis 9:13–16 that He would never destroy the earth by flood, and whenever the rainbow appears in the clouds, He would remember the everlasting covenant between himself and all living creatures of every kind on the earth. The rainbow would be visible when it rains as a sign to all that God will keep His promises. So, God's sign of the rainbow was always my reassurance of His Word and promises—the rainbow reminds me He is there, and He will never leave me nor forsake me.

Still, I longed to be in a flood, because only then would everything be washed away: vanished and gone. Sadly, the rainbow did not come. Most of all, I couldn't *not* see that the sun shining in my room was a sign of the Son, Jesus Christ, reassuring me of His promises.

In my mind, nobody on the outside knew the hell I lived on the inside of my life. Hell is the place I have read about and felt as though I was living, a cold place, a place of darkness where all you see and feel is death. I looked "hell" up many times to see if it was truly a place I wanted to go. At that time in my life, I felt I lived in my personal hell right here on earth, in a depressed state of total suffering every day. I had no control of what would come at me day after day. It was like I had to brace myself for the worst and hope for the best in each minute of the day. I did not know what my mind would be able to handle and how I would be able to separate the dream from the reality. I begged God every day to have mercy upon my soul. I would cry out in agony until I would make myself sick to my stomach. It was such a scary feeling in my mind and my heart that I never want to go back to again. I lay in bed thinking I had nothing to live for; I was stripped of everything in my life. My family beliefs were so strong, and I always said I would never let anything or anyone come between my kids, my family, and me because children are a blessing and a gift from God. Yet, I felt robbed and cheated of my life and my happiness because of this illness. I wanted to die and did not want anyone to find me. I wanted to disappear and die in all of the agony and these uncontrollable tears. I felt my children were better off being raised by my husband, my mother, and their aunts. I was so afraid I would become a vegetable and a burden to everyone. I could not take care of myself, and what kind of mother or wife would I be to my family? They deserved so much better than what I could give them; they were innocent babies who needed a mother's love that I could not give at this time in my life.

My mind was close to being disconnected with the world around me. I wanted to go into hiding until this was all over. Have you ever felt like your life was a movie that you would never want to experience, something you see on television, not ever thinking you could one day be the main character?

I would look around and see all the things that reminded me of a happy home and a wonderful family. My husband, the kids, and I always took family portraits every year, and we would always have different pictures of place we had traveled. There were so many pictures that we had to put them in plastic tubs because we ran out of albums. We did our best to capture every moment of life. These pictures were in our home to remind us of what a blessed family we were. Even the furniture we picked out together was meaningful to both of us because each piece was chosen together in love, just like the colors painted in each room. When we painted our living room, we chose mauve and burgundy, our wedding colors. We painted our bedroom lavender, white, and purple, because it reminded us of royalty and the love we had for Jesus and the love we have for each other. I would think about how my life was so wonderful at one time and how I was so happy. Then, out of nowhere, a giant volcano appeared and erupted with me in the center. There was no way out for me; no matter how much I screamed and grasped for help, I felt like I slowly sunk lower and lower into this massive hole of darkness and despair. I felt like I was spinning in a hellish atmosphere here on earth, but the Lord never let me singe or burn from the heat.

The volcano became a safe haven for me. The medicines kept my mind spinning so much every day until it felt like a whirlpool. I tried to pull myself up, rock by rock, to escape, but I quickly realized there was no escape. I wanted to slowly burn until I turned to ashes so that no one would be able to identify me. There was no one with me where I was, and I couldn't figure out how to climb out of this hole I was slowly sinking down in further and further.

I often got up, went to the window, and looked out, wondering, *Will I ever feel normal again? When will all of this change?* Again, I would ask myself, *Why is this happening to me?*

What was my life going to be like? Everything was too much to handle. I just dwelled every day on the dark feelings in my mind and the painful thought of never being able to raise my children. I would get up in the morning before my husband would leave for work so he could give me my morning dosage of medications before he left. Then he would leave the afternoon doses on the table with a note for me of what to take.

After my husband would leave for work, I would make my way back upstairs and sit on the side of the bed. I had a little blue stool that once belonged to my eight-year-old daughter. I would prop my feet up on that stool, and I would put my hands over my ears and scream as loud as I could and cry out to the Lord, asking Him to please have mercy upon my soul.

I would scream so loud, but I always felt like no one heard me. If I couldn't hear myself, then no one else could hear me. Yet, there I was, screaming and crying, tearing at my clothes because I had lost my mind in my own home. I wanted everything to be over.

I could see myself in a forest with tall trees, and green everywhere in this forest. The sun shone so bright through all of these trees. It was scary to me. These trees were tall—not like any trees I had seen before. It was as though they touched the sky. The trunks, being so richly brown, were striped and swayed back and forth as if a calm wind blew them from side to side. Every time I would look up at them, again, there was the sun, shining so bright that it never appeared to move from that one spot no matter where I turned. I felt like the sun followed me, and I didn't know why. Yet, everywhere I would run, the forest appeared to grow bigger and bigger. I was left with no way out. Yet, there was a beauty in the midst of it all. I always loved being in the sun as a child and even as I grew older. It beamed onto the trees so bright until it looked as though the trees were made of crystal on the top of its leaves. Yet, it scared me because I ran to each part of the forest that I thought was an escape, but each opening was blocked by these huge trees and their distinguished trunks. There, the sun would constantly be right behind me or in front of me. I could not see and realized, once again, the sun that followed me was the Son, Jesus Christ, wanting to rescue and save me. Yet, I was too sick in my mind, body, and spirit to realize that.

As I walked through the darkness confused, scared, and lonely in all the painful places in my life, it was His grace that carried me and His glory He tried to show me. I believe God knew I would not be able to comprehend at that time in my life what He had done for me and through me.

The righteous cry out, and the Lord hears them;
he delivers them from all their troubles.
The Lord is close to the brokenhearted and saves those
who are crushed in spirit.
(Psalm 34: 17-18)

Chapter 5

WANTING TO DIE

I felt as if I slowly died a horrible death in my mind and in my heart.

In the mornings, a shadow would often appear suddenly at my bedroom door. This was always the shadow of a person in a black hooded trench coat. It would speak to me in my mind so plainly and felt as though it spoke directly in my ear, even though it was in the doorway of my bedroom.

This shadow would tell me, "You have nothing to live for; your God has stripped you of everything. Why don't you just kill yourself? You don't look the same. All of your hair is gone, and you don't have your children. Why do you want to live?"

When your mind is already in a delicate place, and the huge amounts of medications (along with their side effects) can cause such a horrific effect, it doesn't take much for the negative thoughts and voices you hear in your mind to convince you to take your life. The voice was deep with a loud piercing echo; I never saw the face because everything about this creature was black.

I began to call this creature Satan. He would tell me, "God has stripped you of everything; you are just like Job."

There I was, trying to figure out in my mind if this was real or if I had truly lost my mind. I was convinced after a short period of time that I should take my life because my life had become worse than I could ever imagine.

One morning in August, after my husband left for work, the devil began speaking to me again reminding me of all that I had gone through and that I had nothing to live for.

I walked downstairs to take my morning medicines by myself; by this time my husband felt I was strong enough to take my thirty pills throughout the day on my own.

I guess I had us both fooled.

I remember standing at the table, crying and screaming, crying out to the Lord, asking Him to help me. I could not decipher the voices that I heard in my mind.

I screamed at the top of my lungs. I was suffocating in my mind. I couldn't breathe. I pulled at what little hair I had left.

I went in the bathroom and looked at myself. My face was still covered with these ugly black lesions all over and a red rash that would not heal because of the severity of the lupus. These lesions were filled with pus and fluid. I looked like someone had just thrown a bag of hot gravel in my face that left me full of burn marks. It was like the aftermath of coming out of the volcano.

The more I looked at myself, the more I screamed uncontrollably and wanted to die.

My face was large, swollen, and round from the ninety-five milligrams of prednisone I had to take each day. My stomach looked as though I was still pregnant.

What was there to live for? To me, there was nothing left of my life.

I was exhausted in my mind and my body. Death was calling me, and I wanted to go. I made my way back into the kitchen, crying out, hoping someone would save me and take this all away.

It felt as though the more I screamed, pulling at my hair and my clothes, the more I sank into a pit of death.

I poured all of my medicines on the table, not just the ones for the morning, but all thirty of them.

The devil told me I had a choice between the pills and any one of the sharp knives. I went to the knife rack on my kitchen counter. Satan's voice was nothing like I had never heard before. His voice was deep, low, and moaning. It was like a deep growl of an old hound that came down deep from his throat, which horrified me. Though it was scary, it was almost hypnotic. He knew how to get into my mind. It was like someone charming you into doing something that you know you do not want to do. The way he said it, it was as if he tried to persuade me. He tried to show me what was best for me and that taking my life was my only option. I felt like his voice had me under a spell. I was so mesmerized by what he said and how he sounded until I could hear nothing else but him.

All I could do was think about was what would be the easiest way. Even though I knew from growing up in the Word of God that Satan comes to kill, steal, and destroy, he had total control of me and mind that morning.

I would ask myself if the pills would take longer to end my life, but I knew the knife would be the fastest and the quickest, so I chose the longest and sharpest knife that I saw.

I wanted to stab the knife through my heart because it hurt so badly. I wanted to rip it out. I wanted die, and that's all that I knew.

I was afraid, but I felt like I had no other choice. As I cried and screamed out, Satan would tell me in one ear to take the pills and to take all of them. Satan also said, "Put the knife in your heart; you have nothing else to live for."

As I stood there cold as ice, my mind felt frozen. I looked around the room and began to think of all the memories that were once in this happy home. I began to clasp my hands over my ears because this demonic voice still pounded these words in my ear to kill myself. The voice began to get heavier and stronger as though he were right in front of me.

Suddenly, from what felt like nowhere, God spoke to me in my other ear, and I could hear His voice so plainly telling me, "You will be all right."

His voice was so peaceful and so calm. It was a voice of assurance. I could feel the gentleness; it was a feeling like being cradled in the arms of my mother. Because God is all-knowing, I believed

He knew how much I wanted and needed my mother to be there to hold me and to rock me, so He began to soothe my heart, taking in all of my emotions and pain. In my mind, I imagined resting in His arms as he held me and rocked me to let me know, "I am here."

For that moment, I felt like a baby, my mother's baby, and it reminded me of how my newborn must feel without her mother's touch.

God spoke to me to tell me how much He loved me and how He would walk with me through this fire.

Yet, though I felt His presence and the presence of the Holy Spirit, I could not, for some reason, grasp everything he said to me, because Satan's voice was so powerful and strong because of the dark place I was in inside my mind.

While everything around me was empty in my mind, life for me was cold, dark, and black. There I was, still screaming and crying while standing at the kitchen table in my nightgown. My hair that I had left on my head was barely combed, and I had not done anything to groom myself for the morning.

The floor felt cold because I had taken off my socks and my slippers. I wanted to die, and I didn't care if they found me or how they would find me.

As I began to look at the pills, I started picking them up, at least six at a time. I kept thinking to myself, *these are so big. Will they all go down? And how soon would they work?* As I began placing them in my mouth, I remembered I had no water, so I took them from my mouth and placed them in my hand. I still held on to the knife with a piercing grip, anticipating using it.

As I walked toward the sink to get a glass of water, still in a fog of confusion and loneliness, I felt like I was in a strange place. I didn't recognize where I was; I slowly moved through the motions of death.

I began talking to myself and telling myself, *I love my baby, I love my daughter, and I love my husband. Yet, I could never be whole again as a mother or a wife. I want to die. What good would I be to anyone?*

In my moment of dark despair and deep depression, the phone rang, and on the answering machine was my husband. As he talked,

I picked up the phone and he said, "I wanted to call to see if you were okay."

He said, "I had this funny feeling and something told me to call you. Did you take your medications for the morning?"

There was a silence on the phone between us, and I began to scream and cry, telling him to help me because I was losing my mind. I dropped the knife on the floor, and I began crying uncontrollably into the phone. All I could hear him say was, "I am on my way home; it's going to be all right. Don't put the phone down. I'm coming home, baby. I'm on my way, and it's going to be all right. Keep talking to me."

But I did put the phone down, and when he arrived home, he found me sitting in the floor, rocking as though my mind was already gone.

My eyes were swollen from all the tears. My gown was ripped because I tried so hard to make it all go away by screaming, crying, and pulling at my body.

I told myself this was the beginning of what I thought would be my end.

He reached down from on high and took hold of me;
he drew me out of deep waters.
He brought me out into a spacious place;
he rescued me because he delighted in me.
(Psalm 18:16, 19)

Chapter 6

UNDERSTANDING
MY DIAGNOSIS

As a child, I used to take a blanket outside and spread it out on the grass. I would lie on my back and look up at the sky and all the white fluffy clouds. My mother once said, "If you stare at the clouds long enough, maybe you will see the image of God."

I do believe I eventually saw God. It was a face shaped in the clouds, and it was as though there were eyebrows, eyes, and long hair. I felt like I had an out-of-body experience, which was so amazing that I knew no one would believe me. I told myself, *Now my life is almost perfect; I have just had my first encounter with God.*

Do we ever consider that in this life we can and will experience a loss of a loved one, a severe illness, or even a financial crisis, not just a setback, but a real financial devastation? Though you look up in the sky and think your world is perfect because you feel you have seen God in the clouds, that does not mean you are living in a perfect world that cannot be touched by tragedy. Have you ever visualized your life as a ship sailing along the seas, the sun shining bright and the sky so blue and clear until it looks as though if you look hard enough, you can see heaven? The waves are coming in, and they are so white and pretty. All you see is yourself cruising along, stopping every now and then to rest upon the sandy shores, enjoying the beauty around you. It feels like you have your own little piece of paradise, not even thinking that one day, your ship can not only be tipped but turned upside down.

Well, I'm here to tell you it can happen to any of us. It all happened to me. My husband and I were happily married, and we had purchased a two-level town home in Clinton, Maryland, with three bedrooms and two baths. We had a nice sized back yard for our daughter to play, in and we could entertain our families when they came to visit. I loved that townhouse because I decorated it with everything that we liked. We felt so richly blessed by God and all he had given us. So, we were now ready to continue expanding our family. My husband James and I always wanted to have two children; even though I had a miscarriage before I had my first daughter Michelle, we wanted to try again. After going to see my obstetrician and speaking with him about having a second child, he suggested that I discontinue taking my birth control pills so I could prepare my body for having another child. So, we began praying and believing God would bless us with another child. After coming off of the birth control pills I felt like I was having some side effects from being on them for so long. I noticed when I would be walking my hip would suddenly give out, and I would fall. I also noticed that my legs would ache some with a cramping pain, and I thought it was just from being on the pill for seven years. I contacted my doctor, who said it was nothing to worry about because some people do have side effects after being on the pill for a long length of time and then coming off of it. I found out that I was pregnant with my second child by doing an in-home pregnancy test. I took the test, which came back positive —was pregnant. After eight years, I kind of thought it wouldn't happen but it did.

I immediately contacted my obstetrician to make an appointment to see him, which was a Thursday on October 14, 1993, so I could have my pregnancy confirmed. My obstetrician called and said, "Lillian I have reviewed the bloodwork, and I have exciting news for you and your husband. I can give you a due date of July 2, 1994. It looks as though you may have conceived around October the 9th, but as time goes on I can give you a more accurate date." He then said, "Congratulations. I will be seeing you soon."

We went to visit my family the next evening just to spend some time with them and to enjoy a seafood dinner they had prepared. My mom and my sister had prepared a seafood salad: steamed crab legs and steamed shrimp, along with some corn on the cob, greens, and fried chicken. As we began to sit down to eat and after saying grace, my mom said to each of us, "It is always good to have at least two children; that way one can play with the other."

Then she looked at James and me and said, "Have you all thought about giving Michelle a sister or a brother?"

We looked at each other and James said, "Well, we thought about it."

So, my mom laughed and said, "You don't want to wait too long; you know you're not getting any younger."

I just smiled and said, "You are right."

James and I both chuckled quietly. That's when James said, "It isn't like we haven't been working on it."

Everyone then laughed uncontrollably. As we began to pass the food around, my sister offered me some seafood salad. I told her, "No, thank you I really don't want to eat anything with may-onnaise in it."

She then offered me some crab legs that she had steamed. Once again I gave her an excuse that I did not have a taste for them. She then said, with a chuckle "What is wrong with you? You don't usu-ally turn down seafood, not as much as you love crab legs."

Then my mom looked at me and then she looked at my sisters and said, "Your sister is pregnant, and I can tell because I am her mother, and a mother knows."

Out of the blue, all of my sisters jumped up with excitement and started yelling and congratulating James and me. My mom then said, "I was going to see how long you were going to sit here before you spilled the beans."

They all were happy for me.

As the days went by, we were still in awe about this baby. We had no idea whether it was a boy or a girl, but we were excited and happy. I would get up and go to work every day with joy, even though some mornings I did have morning sickness. We rode public transportation (commuter bus) to Washington DC every day to work, so there were times in the morning when I would try to eat breakfast, but no matter what I ate, it seemed to upset my stomach. So, I always had to keep a plastic bag with me along with a box of saltine crackers. I hoped and prayed by doing this I would not get sick on the bus. I would often try to get a seat in the back so I could be near the bathroom. The traffic would be so congested that it seemed like with every bump we hit, my stomach was doing flips. It was just so frustrating trying to get to work on public transportation and being pregnant. James and I continued with our everyday lives of going to work during the week and picking Michelle up from the babysitter in the evening. Sometimes I would only have to be concerned with fixing dinner for my husband and myself. Michelle would have already eaten her dinner because the babysitter would feed her before we got home. We would often sit with the babysitter who was actually my neighbor who lived two doors down from us. She was just like a mother to me and a grandmother to Michelle. I remember when I was pregnant with Michelle, she told me, "You will never have to worry about a babysitter because I would love to watch her."

I was blessed to have her as a neighbor and a wonderful babysitter.

I always checked my stomach every day for changes in the size of my stomach and anything that I saw that may have looked unusual on my skin to me since it had been so long. I guess I was just paranoid because I had no idea what I was looking for. My appointments were every six weeks and then changed to every other month.

After a while, I began to show, and my body started to experience changes—one of which was discoloration in my urine. I found it tiresome to go to work some mornings, but I continued to work because I wanted to work until it was time to deliver my baby. My doctor often ordered bloodwork to make sure everything went according to schedule and that the baby and I were in good health. I told my husband after one of my visits, "Don't you think it's a little strange that each time I come for my visit the doctor is always ordering extra bloodwork?, If you think back to when I had Michelle, the doctor took extra bloodwork due to my anemia, and he sent me to a hematologist, but they could never figure out what was wrong. He just gave me more iron pills and vitamins."

My husband then said, "Maybe he is just taking some precautions because of your age and the length of time between your pregnancies."

I then said to James, "My feet seem to be swelling more with this pregnancy, and I hope there is nothing wrong that he is not telling me—or does he suspect something wrong because of my bloodwork results from my last pregnancy?"

James said, "If something was wrong, you would know by now."

I disagreed. My mind just went all over the place, and James, becoming frustrated said, "Look, no news is good news, and let's just leave it at that for now."

After one of my next visits, my obstetrician said, "Mrs. Forbes you are starting to swell more than normal in your feet and ankles. I want you to rest your feet as often as you can."

I had to also keep reminding myself that it had been eight years since I had given birth. I was now thirty-six, so things might be different. After leaving the doctor's office I came home and called my mom to tell her what the doctor had said.

My mother then told me, "Listen to the doctor. If you have to stop working, then you just have to stop working for right now."

My husband and I began preparing for this new addition to our family, and Michelle was so excited to have a little baby brother or sister. She loved to rub my stomach and talk to the baby. We liked to grab one of her storybooks and read it to the baby. We told this little angel that she was coming into a wonderful family who would love her so much, and we were all ecstatic waiting for her arrival. I called the baby a "she," not knowing if it would be a boy or a girl, only because I wanted to have another little girl for Michelle.

We began searching for a crib and different little things to make a nursery special for our little newcomer. Not knowing what we were going to have, we decided to purchase a white Jenny Lynn crib that would work regardless of the sex, and we knew we could not go wrong with white. We purchased mobiles to hang from the crib and pictures with bright rainbows and angels in white frames to match the crib. I bought a little white lamb stuffed animal with curly fur on its body and little pink ears stuck out from the side of his face with an orange and yellow jumpsuit. I placed the lamb in the crib so when the baby came, that was the first thing I wanted her to see. Lambs are considered pure, and a newborn baby is pure and innocent, just like that lamb. We did not paint because the room was already pink, and we all agreed she would be sharing a room with her big sister. We never gave any thought about what we would do with the room if it were a boy.

I continued going to my appointments as scheduled, and I would receive great checkups from my doctor as though everything was going well as far as he could see from examining me. He continued to do the bloodwork, and he kept stressing to me to drink more water. He noticed my red blood cell count was a little low. He became concerned and said he would keep an eye on things as time progressed to make sure everything was okay. I remember still asking James, "Why is he still doing all this bloodwork? Doesn't it seem odd to you by now?" James just quietly smiled and said, "You are fine."

As the weeks and months went by, I noticed small things changing in my body that I never paid much attention to. These changes were different from the symptoms I experienced during my first pregnancy. I noticed my skin was darker than usual; I also began to get extra moles and rashes on my skin. Some of these symptoms did seem a little odd to me. I began to notice the area across the bridge of my nose and cheeks were lighter—not darker—and it was considerably noticeable. I thought the pigmentation in my skin changed because of the hormones.

Then, one day I looked at my face and noticed an unusually shaped flesh mole on the right side of my cheekbone. It was dark brown in color, protruding out of my skin, looking like an oval shape, like a small football, and it always itched. I began picking at it to see exactly what it was, and as I picked at it, it fell off my face. Underneath that mole was white flesh, which I thought was strange because the area from which it had fallen began to burn and sting, but it never bled. It startled me, and I began watching it to see if my skin would come back, and over time, the spot began to close, but it left a dark mark. I shared it with my husband but I never mentioned it to my doctor because I thought my body was just going through pregnancy changes. I wondered why it happened, and when the mole fell off and my skin was burning, I started to wonder what was going on with my skin. I began to think about the extra blood-work that my doctor was taking, and I started to worry.

When I came home after working an eight-hour day, riding the commuter bus back and forth in the morning and the evening my body was tired, and my ankles swelled more and more. Once I got in the house, I would do as the doctor told me and go upstairs to my room and prop up my feet on a stool to stay off them as much as possible. They were so swollen they looked as though they would pop open. I knew eventually my doctor would tell me I would have to stop work earlier than I wanted.

I began to feel more fatigued than usual. I would try not to worry myself with all of the things I experienced in my body, by saying to myself, "You are not a doctor, and all of this is just a part of the pregnancy."

When I was in my seventh month, my doctor started doing urine tests every three weeks to check and see what would be causing me to have so much swelling. He also checked for kidney infections, dehydration, and gestational diabetes. My doctor said all of these tests were precautionary, and he wanted to make sure my urine was clear. He also wanted to be sure that the swelling was not kidney related. Unfortunately, I began to notice my urine output decrease at times. Some months it was clear, and I passed a lot of urine, but other months it was cloudy and felt like less. I constantly drank a lot of water as I hoped it would change the color of my urine. My urine began to turn dark in color, and it was then I became concerned. I talked to my husband and shared with him what was going on with my body. However, in my mind, this pregnancy did not feel like my first one. I knew my body was older, but still something didn't feel right because each time I went to the bathroom, I felt like something was wrong. It was though I had a mother's intuition that something was not right, but I did not know what it was. Whatever it was, I did not want to know. As much as my mind tried to concentrate on having a healthy baby, I could not focus on that. One of the most horrifying thoughts that came to my mind was, *Am I carrying a dead fetus inside me? Is this why my urine has turned so dark? Maybe my doctor does not want to tell me. Is this baby going to be seriously ill with some type of disease?*

On my next appointment with my doctor, he said, "Mrs. Forbes, I think you need to consider stopping work because your feet are not getting any better."

He also said, "I am going to order some more lab work because I am not seeing a change in your urine or your blood. Your urine has become too dark, and that is a great concern for you and the baby. I will see you in one week, and we will order the test, and in the meantime, I want you to prepare yourself to stop work, stay off your feet as much as possible, and please take your vitamins."

I talked with my family and my husband's family, sharing all of the concerns with them that my doctor had shared with us. I had called my mom after one of my visits to tell her what the doctor said concerning my swelling, and she told me to listen to the doctor. When I left the doctor's office, I came home and called my mom again, and I began to share my feelings with her because I wanted her to tell me everything would be okay because by this time, I was concerned. My mother told me to do just what the doctors tell me to do and not have a hard head: stay off my feet and rest myself. She would assure me that everything was fine. It is so comforting when your mother tells you everything is going to be all right; it's a peaceful reassurance that only a mother can give. Still, that did not change the scary feeling of not knowing if anything was wrong. Isn't it strange how you can talk yourself into something, even though you know that is not how you feel on the inside?

By this time, my mind began playing tricks on me with all kinds of thoughts. *Maybe the baby was not going to be healthy.* Or, *something may be wrong with me.* As the weekend went by, I began thinking about everything the doctor had told me, and I began to ask myself, *Is this baby okay? How can I stop work early because we did not plan this part of the journey?*

My sick leave was low, along with my annual leave, so I knew there would be times when my paycheck would not be so great, and I would eventually have to be on leave without pay.

That following Monday, May 16, 1994, when I returned to work, I called my supervisor on the phone to ask her if I could meet with her in the afternoon to discuss my time off from work for maternity leave. She said, "Absolutely, we can meet after lunch around 2:00 P.M."

When it was time to go into the meeting, my heart began to beat harder because I did not know what I was going to tell her or how long I thought I would be away from work. All I could think about was, "What if something is really wrong with me or this baby?"

I knew I did not have any leave, and how would we survive with a sick baby or a sick wife, or even no baby and one paycheck coming in? I eventually got up from my desk and went into the office to have the meeting with my supervisor. I told her, "I don't know where to begin because I know that both my sick and annual leave is low. But I need to let you know that I will need to go on maternity leave earlier than I had anticipated."

I quietly sat there not knowing what her response would be. Before I gave her an opportunity to speak, I just blurted out, "My doctor is concerned with all the excessive swelling, along with my bloodwork."

At this point, my supervisor could see that I was getting emotional. I quickly told her, "I do not want to go into a lot of detail because I don't have much to tell you."

There was so much silence in the room that seemed to go on forever. As the silence broke, I sat there still not knowing what she would finally say.

My supervisor leaned forward and quietly said, "Lillian, I understand, and I have noticed the excessive swelling in your feet. I am not a doctor, but I have also been concerned about what else I have been seeing. I have also noticed a change in your complexion and that you are extremely tired. Let's bring your leave chart up on the computer while you are in here, and we can go from there."

Our conversation then became more administrative. She stated, "As far as your requesting to leave early for maternity reasons, I am reviewing your leave, and you will have to take into consideration the fact that your sick leave and annual leave will all be depleted soon, and you will not have enough to cover your entire time off."

I told my supervisor, with tears in my eyes, "I understand what you are telling me concerning my leave. I really appreciate you meeting with me, but this is something that I did not expect, and I feel like I have no choice because of what my doctor has said."

She then said, "Lillian, I do understand. Your coworkers also want the best for you and your baby."

I got up from my chair and thanked her again, and I said to her, "I will have to pray that the finances work out."

My last day at work was Friday, May 20, 1994. My office wanted to have a baby shower for me, but because my leaving was so abrupt, they did not have time to plan a shower, so they said they would send a gift by James. That was a bittersweet moment for me because I did not have much time to say goodbye to my friends and see a lot of others before I left. I had no idea how long I would be out. I remember crying that day because I did not want to leave early, but still, in my mind, I was afraid something was wrong.

During the week of May 22, I was at home resting and preparing my mind mentally for this new baby. It was hard to stay focused on the everyday things of life because my thoughts were so drawn to what might be happening in my body and to this baby. I went to visit my mom earlier during the week even though I was told to stay off of my feet. I had to see her, and I told her I thought something was wrong, even though the doctors had not yet told me anything. She told me I was going to be fine. It was important for me to see her that week because I had an odd feeling I thought it would be a long time before I would see her again.

Knowing I had a doctor appointment that week, I still had to get Michelle from the babysitter during the day. The babysitter would call me to say Michelle was home from school and she would be sending her over. I would get up to go to the door to let her in and tell her she could have a snack until her daddy came home. She stayed inside until James came, and then he would take her out to play for a little while.

James and I went on as a normal family, doing things that needed to be done in the home and with Michelle. We made sure her homework was done and she was prepared for school every morning. There was not much I could do in the house during that week, but there were times when I was determined to do something, so I would attempt to do some cleaning. James made all the trips to the grocery store and other errands that needed to be done. He would get Michelle up in the morning, fix her some cereal, and made sure she bathed. I managed to help her lay her clothes out at night so everything would not fall on my husband. I styled her hair at night with the style she liked: bangs and two pigtails on the side with hair barrettes. And I would tie her hair up with a scarf so we would not have to comb it in the morning.

Before James walked her over to the babysitter, she would come into my bedroom and say, "Mommy, I love you," and kiss my stomach and say, "That is for my little sister."

We continually told her that we didn't know if she would have a little sister or a little brother because we did not want to know the sex of the baby.

My next appointment was scheduled for Friday May 27, 1994 at 4:00 P.M. On that day, as I prepared to go to my appointment, Michelle was with the babysitter. For some reason, I felt something strange in my heart, but I just could not figure out what it was. I was anxious and fidgety, but I tried to think about other things that I would have to do once the baby came, and we were even talking about how we never even discussed a name. For some reason, I still felt something in my gut that something was happening inside my body, and I did not know what it was. Have you ever been so nervous and irritable that the least little question asked bothered you? That's exactly how I felt. My husband asked me something, and I would snap back at him because I dwelled on what could possibly be wrong with me.

Once we arrived at the doctor's office, I was even hesitant to get out of the car, so my husband said, "Let's pray and go hear what the doctor has to say, and we will go from there. I am sure that everything is going to be fine."

I walked as slow as I could, not only because my feet hurt, but I was not thrilled about going in the office. After waiting for an hour and a half past my scheduled appointment time, the nurse walked over to me and said, "Mr. and Mrs. Forbes, the doctor will see you both now."

I was upset, so I asked, "Why did they give me that appointment time to make me wait for an hour and a half before I was seen?"

She said, "The doctor would like to talk with you and your husband and that is the reason he wanted to see you both last."

As we both headed back into the doctor's office, he greeted us both at the door with a smile and a handshake. I could see concern in his eyes. I sat in the chair next to the window while my husband sat in the chair directly in front of the doctor's desk. My doctor sat at his desk, twirling his pencil, looking at us both with hesitation and a stone look on his face. It was like someone had something shocking to tell you but they did not know what the best way would be to say it. So, he said, "Mr. and Mrs. Forbes, I do apologize for the wait but I needed this time so I could talk with you and your wife concerning her bloodwork that I have received."

He then said to us, "As you both know, I have been ordering extra bloodwork and monitoring Lillian's urine output and her excessive swelling."

While he was talking, he continued to also look down at my medical file, still with hesitation. All of a sudden, my mouth became dry, and I had a big lump in my throat, as though I had tried to swallow a large ball that would not go down. No matter how much I tried to swallow this ball, it kept getting stuck in my throat. I felt like I choked on silence. My focus had left me, I started to feel numb, and the doctor had not begun to say anything yet. I felt nervous and my teeth itched and my heart felt like it raced a mile a minute. All I could do was look at the expression on his face and see that whatever he had to say, he found it difficult to do. It was an expression of sadness, though he knew he had to share with us the results of the lab work. I didn't know if it was something about the baby or me. Finally, after watching the doctor open my medical file and clearing his throat, I sat there hoping that the chair I was sitting in would not hold me. I was really scared. At that moment,

I wanted to go through the floor—just disappear—because I had no idea what he was going to say. Suddenly, he sat up sternly in his chair and took his glasses off, put his pencil down, and said, "Mrs. Forbes, I don't want you to upset you with what I'm going to tell you and your husband. But I have some serious concerns about your pregnancy, and I need to discuss this with you both. Because of the fact that you are so far along in your pregnancy, this has me greatly concerned."

He reached for his glasses again as he began to read my test results and told us, "I received your bloodwork, and I see where you have a large amount of protein in your urine that is spilling from your kidneys. This protein spill causes the urine to become dark. This is not healthy for you or your unborn baby."

He then said, "The amount you are spilling is 500 grams a day, which is dangerous. This is a serious matter, and we have to act now in doing everything we can to protect the kidney, Lillian, and this baby."

As soon as he mentioned the word "kidney" again, I wanted to sink right through the chair; it was though that set off an alarm in my mind. I remember my eyes filled up with water and the tears were hard to hold back. When I hear something about the kidneys, the first thing that comes to mind is something devastating, something so catastrophic it cannot be fixed.

As he tried to explain to my husband how the kidney works and the damage that protein in the urine can cause, I could hear my husband asking questions. My husband said to the doctor, "I don't know much about the kidneys, but I understand enough to know that the kidney is a vital organ that removes waste products and excess fluid from the body which is passed through the urine. What I don't understand is how protein plays a part in this? What I would like to know is, what can we do to stop the urine from spilling protein from her kidneys and what can be causing this?"

The doctor then said, "Mr. Forbes, you are correct in your assessment of what the kidney does." As my husband tried to be strong for the both of us, my mind was lost in space. I looked out the window in the parking lot, watching people get in and out of their cars. I couldn't listen to anything the doctor said, and I completely blocked out everything as I sat in that chair. I could hear him, but my body and mind were not present.

Then, he proceeded to say, "I think she may have this chronic disease called lupus. I am not certain, but I would like to send her to Georgetown University Hospital as soon as she can go to have further testing done. A weekend day would be better because they would be able to do the test right away."

Before the doctor could finish explaining what he wanted us to do, my husband interjected again and said, "Lupus? Doctor, I have heard of this disease, but I do not know much about it; how serious is this? I have heard of people passing away from this disease. How do you get this, and is this something that is hereditary?"

The doctor then said to my husband, "No gene has been proven to cause lupus; however lupus does appear in certain families, and it affects the immune system which is the part of the body that fights off viruses and bacteria. The cause for lupus in most cases is unknown, and the symptoms vary from person to person."

The doctor went on to say, "We will need to do several more blood tests, along with an amniocentesis to see how far the baby has developed since you are in your eighth month of pregnancy."

He also said, "You will just have to go there for one day, on Saturday May 28, 1994, for these tests, and you will be able to come back home. It may take several hours to get the results back, so you may be there for several hours. So just prepare yourself an overnight bag just in case it may take longer. I will contact the hospital to arrange everything to let them know that you will be coming."

I sat in the chair, cold as ice. It felt as though I stood in the street and a big steamroller had come by and flattened me to the pavement. It was as if I had no physical feeling left in me. I could not feel any emotion, and I felt paralyzed in my brain. I could not believe what I heard. Finally, the tears rolled down my face as I still cried in silence. I could hear my husband keep asking me if I was okay and if I listened to what the doctor said. All I could do was continue to look out the window. It was as though something drew me to the outside, where I would not be able to hear anything that

47

was said. That is just how much I wanted to run out of that office. I could not grasp the reality of the news I heard that day.

As I continued to look out the window, I was mesmerized, thinking I was in a dream. I tried to count the leaves on the trees to distinguish how many were orange, red, or purple—anything to take my mind somewhere else. The strangest thing is, as I got to the seventh leaf while counting in my mind, I could hear this soft, still voice speaking in my ear like a whisper.

When the doctor or my husband spoke, it was as though I could not hear them, but this small, quiet, still voice whispered so gently in my right ear, almost pulling my ear up so I could hear.

This voice said to me, "Your life is going to change."

I did not understand it, because when that was spoken to me, I thought that I would have to take some pills and everything would be okay.

After we agreed to go to Georgetown to take these special tests and as I got up to leave, my body felt paralyzed, and it was as though I was a zombie going through the motions. I remember looking in the doctor's eyes as the tears continually rolled down my face. I had no questions to ask, and I knew there should have been many, but my mind and my heart were in disbelief. All I wanted to do was run somewhere and scream. I couldn't because I had this little life inside of me.

As we left his office, I remember the doctor looking at me and my husband as he put his hand on my husband's shoulder. The doctor then asked us, "Are you guys okay? I am sorry for what I had to tell you."

I felt a sigh of relief for that moment as though I was being consoled by my doctor. Getting in the elevator, and going to the car, I did not look at my husband. I did not want to hear anything he had to say. Though I knew it was not his fault, I wanted to blame whoever I could.

As we drove home, I put my face in my hands and cried until I felt drained. The tears I cried that I could not let out in the doctor's office soon exploded when I was somewhere I could let go. Riding home, I was silent, but I could still here that still, small voice saying to me, "Your life is going to change."

As we pulled up to the babysitter's house to get Michelle, my husband said, "I need you to try to get yourself together because Michelle is going to know something is wrong."

I said to my husband, "I just can't understand why this is happening to me. Tell me this is bad dream and that I'm going to wake up from it."

My husband said "I know this is shocking and it hurts; believe me, I hurt with you, but we can't let Michelle see us upset."

As we got out of the car and went into the babysitter's house, my girlfriend was there also picking up her son. She came over to me with excitement and hugged me with a big smile on her face and said "Lil, how are you? And how did your appointment go?"

She was more excited than I was, but before I could answer her she could tell something was wrong by the expression on my face. It was an expression of deep concern and sadness. I said, "I'm fine," but my eyes were filling up with tears. She stood there with tears in her eyes as she continued to stare at me and see that I was beginning to cry. She said, "You know that I am here if you want to talk. I don't know what's wrong, but I know everything will be okay."

The babysitter told her daughter to take the kids in the other room so she could talk with my husband and me. She then asked me with a concerned look on her face, "Lil, how did your doctor's appointment go?"

All I could do was burst loudly into tears. My husband, while his arm was around me, quickly told the babysitter, "Lil has to go to Georgetown on Saturday for some special tests."

The babysitter then said, "James, you and Lil come and sit down and tell me what's going on and tell me what the doctor has said."

As we all began to sit down, I was crying a little louder by this time. James said to the babysitter and my girlfriend, "The doctor thinks Lil has this chronic disease called lupus."

All off a sudden there was silence in the room, and my babysitter said, "We are going to pray right now. I want all of us to pray asking God to touch Lil and this precious little baby in the name of Jesus."

After we finished praying, they kept trying to reassure us that everything was going to be okay.

After sitting with my babysitter for a while, we finally gathered Michelle's things and went home. We did not have to feed her dinner because she had already eaten at the babysitter's house. Before we did anything, we took a deep breath as we looked at each other and we sat Michelle down between the both of us. I then said to her, "Mommy and Daddy need to talk with you about something important."

Michelle, being the sweet little eight-year-old that she was said, "Okay, Mommy, I'm listening."

I started off by asking, "How was your day at school?"

Michelle said, "Mommy, it was okay. Guess what? I told my teacher that my little sister or brother is coming, and I'm going to be the babysitter."

I looked at Michelle and smiled and said, "Mommy loves you." James then said, "Michelle, Mommy needs to go to the hospital for some special tests this weekend, so how would you like to spend the weekend with Granny until Mommy comes back home?"

I sat there trying not to cry trying to reassure her that I would only be gone for one day. I said, "Michelle I will be back home before you have to go back to school on Monday."

Michelle looked up at me and then she looked at her dad with those big brown eyes and said, "Mommy, are you really okay? Is my little sister okay?"

She sat there slowly rubbing my stomach in a circle. James rubbed her cheek and said to her, "Your mommy and your little sister are fine, but the doctor has to do some extra things to make sure."

Michelle looked up at both of us and said, "Mommy, I love you, and Daddy, I love you too."

Then Michelle laid her head and ear on my stomach and said, "Little Baby Sister, I love you too."

I sat there trying my best for her not to see me cry while I just looked at that little innocent face. I could not tell her about the uncertainty that I was feeling on the inside.

She then asked me, "When will I be going to Granny's house?"

I smiled at her and said, "As soon as you come home from school tomorrow evening."

Then James took her downstairs to watch television. I then made a phone call to my mom and said, "I want to tell you some of what the doctor told James and I today."

But as soon as I began talking my voice started to crack, and I told her I would call her back. I had to get off the phone and cry. While Michelle was still watching television, I called James and asked him to please come upstairs. I said to him through my sobs, "I can't get myself together, I'm trying, but I just can't. So, could you please call my mother back and tell her what's going on."

James called my mother and told her, "I will explain everything in more detail once we arrive on Friday, because I do not want Michelle to hear me talking."

We finally got to my mom's about eight o'clock on Friday evening. James and I talked with her and my sisters to let them know I would only be there for several hours on Saturday and that he would be back to get Michelle on Sunday evening. He wanted to bring her home so she could prepare for school. We stayed there until 10:30 P.M. talking and eating with everyone.

Finally, James said, "We have to leave in order to get some rest and make an early start for the morning." We told my mom that we would call her after everything was done and we were headed home. Michelle was still up and playing with some of her cousins. She kissed us goodnight and hugged us both. It made me feel better knowing she was okay with being away from me for a little while. When James and I got home, we began to talk about what was going on and how we would be strong and try to handle the situation. As I packed my bag, I only packed enough for overnight because that was how long I intended on staying, according to the doctor.

That night, I could not sleep. I tossed and turned all night because my mind couldn't stop imagining what was going on and what these tests would show. The next morning, which was Saturday, we got up and got dressed and proceeded downtown to Washington DC to Georgetown Hospital. We arrived at the hospital at 9:30 A.M. and checked in with the receptionist, who directed us to where we needed to go. Once I was there, the doctor and nurse came out to talk with us, letting us know exactly what test they would be doing that morning and how I would be able to go home that same evening. The nurses came back out into the waiting area about ten, and they took me into an office. One of the nurses began to go over different procedures the doctor had ordered. She said, "The procedure will be the amniocentesis test and an ultrasound and sonogram." She also said, "When we begin the tests, we will explain them to you in greater detail.

With fear in my eyes, I told her, "I understand."

My husband said, "I am glad you are running these tests because I am concerned."

The nurse also stated, "These tests are being done as a precaution in case we have to do an emergency Cesarean birth because of the lupus."

The two procedures took about an hour to do. My husband waited until all the procedures were done, then the doctors brought me back out around 11:00 A.M. and said we would have to wait for an hour for all of the results to come back. We went to the hospital cafeteria to get something to eat and to kill time until we thought the tests were completed. We were both nervous and scared because we did not know what kind of news to expect to hear.

Around noon, we went back to the area where they did the testing, and the obstetrician was waiting with the nurses to talk with us. The doctor called us both into his office and asked us to please sit down because he and the nurse wanted to discuss the test results from the bloodwork. The nurse asked us both, "Would you like some water or maybe some juice?"

I then told her, "We're fine."

The nurse had a strange look on her face, just like the look my obstetrician had when he gave me bad news. After we told her that we were fine, she never said anything else. She looked at the doctor, and he looked at her. The doctor got straight to the point; he did not beat around the bush. He came out and said, "Mrs. Forbes, the test we took confirmed what your obstetrician had found and we repeated the same test along with other tests we felt would help confirm our findings."

He continued, "Mrs. Forbes, you have lupus and an extremely serious case of it, a case which we have not come across that often in pregnant mothers who are so close to full term. Lupus symptoms can be unclear, and they can come and go. Mrs. Forbes, unlike other chronic illnesses, trying to reach a diagnosis of lupus isn't always easy. However, because of the more extensive tests we ran on you concerning the bloodwork, which shows high amounts of protein that you are spilling, your kidneys are being attacked by this disease."

He went on to say, "Your kidneys are not pumping out the waste in your body that is needed for you while you are carrying this baby. This is why you have so much excessive swelling. Your white blood cell count is low, and that is causing your anemia. Because of all of these symptoms, there is no doubt that you and your baby are at a high medical risk, and we feel that you need to be admitted today until you deliver your baby."

The doctor then explained, "Mrs. Forbes, you are spilling 500 grams of protein a day from your kidney, and this is way too much. The reason so much protein is spilling from your kidneys is because the lupus has attacked one, of your kidneys, and it can get into the other kidney if treatment is not started. We need to start a treatment process as soon as possible because lupus is a complicated disease, and it could eventually attack other organs in your body. Your kidneys can shut down while you are carrying this baby, and it will be harmful for you and your child if we were to start dialysis. We hope that we will not have to go that route. We want to try and turn the lupus around, so you and your baby can survive this." Finally, he said "Mrs. Forbes, the lupus could possibly get in the baby's blood stream and cause a stillbirth."

All I could do once again was cry and sit in shock. The doctor looked at James and me and said, "Mr. Forbes, we would like to admit your wife today because she is so far along in her pregnancy, and we do not want to risk anything more going wrong."

The doctor saw I was crying and upset. He then said, "Mrs. Forbes, this way we can monitor you and your baby. You will receive the best care that we can give you both here at this hospital."

As I finally looked at him all I could say to him was, "But I am not due until July 2 and this is a long time to be in the hospital."

He said, "I understand, but I think we need to do what is best for you and the baby. In the meantime, I will contact your obstetrician and let him know the course of action that we will be taking." The doctor got up from his desk and said, "I will give you two some time alone in case you have questions you need to ask me. My phone is available if you need to call any one."

He left his office, and immediately I looked at James, and he looked at me; we just stared at each other, not saying anything. I knew he tried his best to be strong for me, but the tears rolled down his face along with mine.

James said, "We have to trust God that everything is going to be okay."

I looked at him as though I did not want to hear that, and I immediately said to him, "What about Michelle? She is not going to want to stay at my mom's this whole time."

James then said, "Let's call your mom and tell her what the doctor said and we will go from there." James continued, "Right now I want you to take a deep breath, and try to stay calm, so you won't continue to upset yourself or the baby."

After my husband was able to calm me down, we proceeded to call my mom on the phone. James told her, "The doctor wants Lillian to stay in the hospital, and I will explain everything to you when I see you," telling her, "I don't want to go into detail over the phone."

My mom then said "I understand, and I am keeping you all in prayer."

James reminded her that he would still be coming to get Michelle on Sunday.

My mom said, "I will let you talk to Michelle when you come. James, you need to go home and get some rest, and we will talk tomorrow."

Once the doctor came back into the office, we had several questions we wanted to ask him. The first thing we wanted to know was what would be his method of treatment since I was so far along in the pregnancy. We also wanted to know the type of medication that I would be receiving and how that would affect the baby. Before the doctor began his answers, the first thing he said was, "We would like to go ahead and start the admitting process by having you to fill out the necessary papers, and then I will come to your room and talk with you and your husband."

The nurse came back in with a wheelchair and said, "Mrs. Forbes, we are going to wheel you down to admitting so we can get you admitted to the hospital into a room where you can be comfortable. How are you feeling?"

I did not have an answer for her. All I could do was look down at the floor and go along with everything she said because my mind was in a fog. I had no idea how this happened; all I knew was that I came here for some bloodwork for one day that turned into a month-long stay. I was speechless. Finally, we got to my room, and the nurse said, "I will go talk with the doctor, but in the meantime, I want you to change your clothes and get in the bed off of your feet."

My husband began to help me get undressed and into my nightgown. He helped me to get in the bed and tried to get me comfortable. I was not interested in anything she had to say. I was angry and I was mad—mad at my doctor, mad at the doctors at this hospital, and I began to get upset with my husband.

Once I got into the bed, I tried to ball up in a knot as best as I could because I did not want anyone to say anything to me, and I did not want anyone to touch me. I wanted to be left alone.

My husband sat in the chair beside the bed, still trying to carry on a conversation while trying to rub my feet, but I told him to please stop; I just did not want to be touched. The nurse came back in about forty-five minutes later with the doctor who was my new obstetrician at this hospital.

He said to my husband and me, "I know this is a lot to take in at one time, but I will do my best to answer some of your questions and concerns today, but tomorrow we can talk again."

The first thing that he wanted to do was put me on a fluid pill called Lasix to try to relieve some of the excess fluid from my feet. The second thing he wanted to do was immediately start me on a low dose of prednisone, a mild dose of twenty milligrams. He said that would help stop the protein from spilling from my kidneys, but it would take a few days to get into my system. He never went into anything more except to say they would watch me around the clock because my body was not well—especially being pregnant. So, they started the medications right away.

The doctor said, "We will be taking you down to the endoscopy unit three times a week so we can listen for the baby's heartbeat and check on movement from the baby."

My husband asked the doctor "When doing this endoscopy test, do you ever experience a time when the heartbeat and the movement is slow?"

The doctor said, "Yes, and this is why we want to do the test three times a week." He then proceeded to say, "If the baby is in distress we will know right away.

Also, we will be drawing your blood three to four times a week to keep track of the protein and to see how rapid the lupus is moving. But for right now, I would like for you to get some rest and try not to worry." He also smiled and said, "We will take good care of you and your baby."

My husband walked over to the doctor looked him in the eye, shook his hand, and said, "I really appreciate all that you are doing to make sure my wife and baby are fine."

The doctor then said, "Mr. Forbes, we are going to do our best; the nurse will be bringing you something to eat in a little while and she will come back. She will sit with you and your wife for a few minutes just in case there are other questions you may need to ask." The doctor smiled, rubbed my arm, and said, "I will check on you first thing in the morning as he walked away."

James and I sat together in that hospital room—he was in the chair, and I sat up in the bed. We may have said two or three words to each other from 11:30 A.M. to 4:30 P.M. We were both in our own world trying to take in all of this. Finally, he dozed off, and I would try to fall asleep, but I couldn't. I would stare at him while he tried to sleep, asking myself, "What are we going to do?"

Finally, the nurse came back in with food for my husband and me. She said, "Mr. Forbes, I know you are probably tired and hungry and you have been here since nine-thirty this morning, and it is now five o'clock in the afternoon. So, I brought you something to eat and some coffee also if you would like to have some."

While we ate, the nurse reassured us that everything would be okay, and if I needed her to page the front desk and ask for Rose. She got up from her chair and shook my husband's hand and told him to try not to worry and then she said, "Mrs. Forbes, I will see you in the morning."

I finally spoke a few words to her and said, "Thank you and goodnight."

My husband sat in the chair, still eating some of his food, but he said he didn't have an appetite, but he said, "I want you to please try to eat something."

After he finished his meal and drank his coffee, he said, "I think I need to start heading back down the road, and I will be back here tomorrow morning early, so I will not miss the doctor when he comes in. I will not go to church at all; I will come right here."

I felt sad, not wanting him to leave me, so I began to cry again, and he did everything he could to console me. Finally, I got myself together, and he said, "Call me if you cannot sleep or if anything changes with you during the night. I will be back first thing in the morning, so let me know what you need me to bring you from the house."

As he began to leave, he hugged and kissed me, then he said, "I will call your mom once I am in the car, and I will talk to Michelle when I get there. I still want her to stay with your mom until Sunday evening because I am exhausted, and I want to try to get some rest so I can be here early in the morning. I just don't have the heart to tell Michelle that she would be away from her mommy for a whole month."

After James left, I tried my best to sleep, but my mind wouldn't let me; it felt like a river running in all different directions, steadily going downstream.

When Sunday morning came, I woke up and felt like I had been kidnapped. I felt like I was somewhere I definitely did not want to be and was held against my will. Even though somewhere inside of me, I knew this was something I knew was best for my child and me, I still did not want to be there.

The doctor came into my room, along with two nurses to ask me how I felt. I told them I was tired and I didn't understand how this happened.

The doctor said, "Mrs. Forbes, what I need you to do is just try to relax and let us take care of you and your baby so you both can begin to get better."

The doctor then asked, "Mrs. Forbes is your husband coming up today?"

I told him, "He is on his way."

He then replied, "Once your husband gets here, let the nurse know, and they will have me paged. I'm certain your husband has more questions, and there are some other medications that I will need to start. Also, I would like to discuss these medications with you and your husband together."

The doctor and the nurse then left my room. I called James on the phone and asked, "How soon will you be at the hospital?"

James replied, "I should be there in another twenty minutes."

I then asked him "Did you speak to Michelle last night like you said?"

He said, "I told her I would be getting her Sunday evening and that mommy had to stay an extra day. I did not want to try and explain things to her all at once because I know she would be upset and would not understand."

Finally, James arrived at the hospital and greeted me with a hug and a kiss, but I could still see much concern in his eyes.

The doctor said, "Mr. Forbes, as I have confirmed to you both earlier, your wife is sick with an extremely serious case of lupus."

I could see James staring directly at me.

The doctor then said, "I have been in consultation with her obstetrician, who recommended that she come see me and other colleagues here at the hospital."

He walked closer to the bed and said, "Because of the severity of the lupus and the fact that she is eight months pregnant, it is necessary that we put her on additional medications to try to keep the lupus under control. Doing that will also make a safe delivery for the baby. These medications will help reduce the spill of protein from the kidneys and reduce the fluid buildup in her legs and feet."

Finally, the doctor said, "I have given the nurse the list of medications and we would like to start her on these today. But I want to caution you both that Mrs. Forbes may feel a little different in her body because of the different medications, but we will be keeping a close eye on her."

My husband quickly spoke up and said, "What about the baby? How will these medications affect the baby?"

I wanted to ask that question too, but I could not open my mouth to speak. The doctor reassured us that the medications would not go through the placenta, so the medications should not affect the baby.

He then said, "I will check back with you later this evening to see how you are feeling, so please try to get some rest."

I thought to myself, *How I can possibly get some rest when I feel like I have just run into a brick wall?* As the doctor walked out, the nurse left behind him and said she would be back shortly with the new medications. Once again, James and I did not share a lot of words between us—only space filled the room. Finally, the nurse came back with a long list of medications. I was given furosemide which helped to reduce my fluid buildup in my legs and feet. I was also given Vasotec, which improved the amount of oxygen in my blood and it was to help reduce my blood pressure. The Cozaar and the Prinivil that I was given helped to reduce my blood pressure. Finally, Plaquenil was given to me for the inflammation in my joints.

I looked at the nurse and said to her, "Are you sure this will not affect my baby? Because you have given me three different strong blood pressure medicines, a fluid medicine, and a medicine for my lupus. These are all five additional different medications, which does not include the twenty milligrams of prednisone that you have me on."

The nurse put her hand on my shoulder and said, "Mrs. Forbes, these medicines are what you need to keep your body well and the lupus stable so you can carry your baby full term."

I looked at her with great concern and said, "These are all strong medications. How bad are my side effects going to be?"

The nurse reiterated, "We will be taking good care of you."

I was still worried about the amount of medications.

The nurse then said, "Now that you have had your breakfast, we want you to start taking these right away."

She began to pour me a glass of water and instructed me to take them one at a time. She also said, "You may have some side effects with these, but it is necessary for a healthy baby and a safe delivery."

I looked at my husband with much hesitation in my eyes and he said, "Please take them; I will be right here with you. And if you doze off, it is okay because when you wake up, I will be here by your side."

I began to swallow each pill, one at a time, while the nurse made sure I took them. As she began to walk out, she said, "Someone will be in later this evening to do some bloodwork."

Michelle had to go to school on Monday, and James wanted her to come home, rest, and prepare for school. He left for the evening and said that he would call me later. After he left, the nurse came in to draw my bloodwork that the doctor had ordered and asked me if I needed anything.

I told her I was fine, and then she looked at me and said, "I can see the worry and sadness in your eyes, but it's going to be okay."

I was so tired of everyone telling me it was going to be okay when I was the one not knowing if my baby or I would live or die.

James came by Monday evening and brought me some beautiful roses to cheer me up. The next day, which was Tuesday morning, the nurse came back and said, "We would like to take you down to the endoscopy unit to have your first sonogram this morning."

She and another nurse helped me to get out of bed and in the wheelchair, and they rolled me down a long hallway. When I got in the room, they helped me to get onto a bed with several beeping machines.

The nurse said, "Mrs. Forbes, we will be doing the two tests today that we discussed earlier. One will be an ultrasound /sonogram to check for fetal movement and to look at the placenta. The other test will be an amniocentesis which can show us how far developed the baby's lungs are and to check for any genetic disorder. We just want to make sure that your baby is not in any type of distress."

As I lay there not knowing what to expect from the test, the nurse began to ask me several questions.

"Mrs. Forbes, before I start the test, can you tell me if you have felt much movement or activity with the baby such as kicking over the last several weeks?"

Before I could answer her, she said, "How about since you have been admitted?"

I told her no. I then told her, "I have not felt a lot of movement, and I thought the baby was sleeping."

She then asked me, "Do you know the sex of the baby?"

I told her, "I never wanted my doctor to tell us because we wanted to be surprised. But my daughter, Michelle, wants a little sister."

So, as she began to perform the two tests, she began to rub the cold gel on my stomach, and she said, "I will be doing the ultra sound first, and I will be using a hand-held device called a transducer, and I'll be rubbing all around your abdomen in different areas. This will allow me to observe the fetal movement and to look at your placenta."

During this procedure, she said nothing, but she did look up at me periodically and smile. Still, I saw a concerned look come over her face each time she looked at the screen.

Finally, she broke her silence and said, "Mrs. Forbes, you are having a girl."

I smiled and said to myself, "Thank you God."

Once she finished the first test, she began to gently wipe the gel from my stomach as she began to explain the amniocentesis test to me. "They will be inserting a needle into your womb drawing a small amount of amniotic fluid. This will determine the maturity of the lungs and any possible genetic disorders."

I was still concerned because I felt that the nurse had more to tell me. I was so happy on the inside to know I was having a girl because I knew that's what Michelle wanted—a baby sister. Then reality hit me and the nurse asked, "Why are you looking so sad?"

I told her, "I just want my baby to be healthy. How is the heartbeat? I did not feel any movement when you examined me."

She said, "Don't worry; I do feel a faint heartbeat, and I am going to let the doctor know. The baby is probably just sleeping."

When you pass through the waters, I will be with you;
And when you pass through the rivers, they will not sweep over you.
When you walk through the fire, you will not be burned; the flames will not set you ablaze.
(Isaiah 43:2)

Chapter 7

THE STORM IS HERE

As time went on and the days went by, I lay in that bed wondering what my and my baby's fate would be. James and I finally had to discuss how we would try to work this situation out with Michelle. After a long tearful discussion, we both decided that he would keep Michelle with him. He brought Michelle up to see me twice for a visit, but he would always let her call and talk to me on the phone. I just didn't want her to have the memory of her mom lying in the hospital for such a long time, so we felt it was best to visit twice and to keep in close contact over the phone. As I spoke with James, I could tell that it was hard for him and Michelle.

James said, "I do not want to burden your mother with Michelle staying there all that time while you are in the hospital."

I told James, "It would be too much trouble to take her out of school."

So, we decided that he would get Michelle dressed for school in the morning and take her to the babysitter's house. He had help from the babysitter when it came to doing Michelle's hair and on the weekends, he would take her to my mother's while he tried to get some rest.

My mother and sisters would call me to see how I was doing, but that was not too often because they were helping my mom take care of my dad. I would ask my mom how my dad was doing because I knew he was sick also. James would let Michelle call me before the evening got too late and talk with me before she would go to bed. I would ask her, "Michelle, how was your day at school?"

She would say, "Fine. When are you coming home? Are you bringing my new sister?"

I told her, "Mommy will be coming home soon."

When James came to see me the next day, he asked me, "Is it okay if I let people know that you are going to be in the hospital for a while?"

I told him, "Yes."

One afternoon, after my testing and bloodwork, I returned to my room, and there was a knock at my door. When I said come in, it was my two Bible study instructors and two of our church members. I was so touched by their presence that they thought enough about me to come see me. They stayed with me for an hour, and we talked and had prayer. One of the church members said, "Be encouraged and trust God in knowing that He is with you."

One of my Bible study instructors told me, "I will stay in contact with James to see how you are progressing."

I hugged them all and thanked them for coming. I also thanked them for their prayers.

Besides the Bible study group, James and two of my sisters came to visit me. I received few visitors. That hurt also because I was lonely, and I wanted to know people cared about me. The nurses would come three times a week, as they had said, to take me down for testing. The heartbeat of the baby was still faint, and there was not a lot of movement, but the doctor said he did not want the baby to come too early because he wanted to make sure that the lungs would be fully developed.

One day, while having the sonogram done, the nurse asked, "Mrs. Forbes, have you or your husband chosen a name for your daughter?"

I told her, "Yes we have; her name is Sheree."

She said, "That is a beautiful name. How did you decide upon that name?"

I guess she was making my time there with her pleasant in order to take my mind off the sonogram.

I said, "My husband is a Stevie Wonder fan, and he named her after one of his songs."

She smiled and said, "That is so special."

As she did the sonogram, she would call Sheeree's name to see if she could spark any more movement, but the movement was still not as spontaneous as they wanted it to be.

After my tests, I returned to my room, lay on my back while looking up at the ceiling crying, and said, "God, if you can hear me, please help me because I am tired, and I just don't know what to do."

A few times I would attempt to get up and go to the window just to look at the outside. I had not seen the outside in so long that it was almost as if I forgot how it felt. I would tell God, "I just don't know how much of this I can take, and please don't let my baby die."

Time had passed, and there appeared to be no change in my kidneys, but the blood pressure was stable. The doctors were still concerned with the large amount of protein still spilling from my kidneys. It was so strange because over time, when the doctors came into my room, they would always come in groups of five. This would consist of a team of doctors because Georgetown was a teaching hospital, and they would always include new interns coming into the practice. This particular day, when they came into my room, I was lying there just staring at the wall. Though I carried this baby inside of me, I felt empty and alone. My eyes were red and swollen from so many tears that I had cried. I felt like they were all staring at me as though I was on display. As my main doctor talked and was explaining my illness to the team of doctors that was with him, they looked at me with smiles and concerns. Unfortunately, that did not make me feel any better. My doctor then asked me, "Do you have any questions at all that you would like to ask?"

I dried my tears enough to ask him, "How am I doing, and is there any change in my condition?" The doctor began to explain,

"We will have to increase the prednisone to ninety-five milligrams in order to control the protein from spilling from your kidneys. We will try this for a few days, and then we will do one last ultra sound/sonogram to check for fetal movement and to look at the placenta again."

I said to the doctor, "I'm scared, and I don't know if I can handle any more of this."

The doctor said, "Mrs. Forbes, I know you are afraid and have great concern, but please try not to worry."

Then the doctor, with a look of sensitivity on his face, trying to reassure me, said, "We will not do another amniocentesis because at this far along in your pregnancy the ultrasound will show us if we need to deliver the baby immediately."

After the doctor finished talking, I thought to myself, *This all sounds like foreign language to me that I do not understand.* I immediately asked him, "Will this high dose of prednisone harm my baby?"

The doctor assured me again, "You and the baby will be fine."

However, in my mind, I always believed that while you are carrying a child you should not be taking large dosages of medication because you could harm the fetus. The doctor could see the great concern in my eyes and on my face, so he said, "If the lungs are fully developed, we will be doing an emergency cesarean birth. We are trying to hold out as long as we can, but things are beginning to get crucial for you and the baby."

I remember the doctor looking me directly in my eyes and saying, "Unless God works a miracle, you could possibly die and the baby would probably not survive because of the severity of the lupus."

I began to get terrified; I was not ready to die, and I did not want my baby to die. I was ready for everything to be over with because all of the medicines were making me so delirious in my mind that I could not think clearly. When my husband came to see me that evening, he noticed that I was quiet, more so than usual. James began to start his conversation by saying, "Everyone at work has been asking about you, and I have been receiving so many cards in the mail."

I felt as though he was trying to avoid what he wanted to talk about. Finally, he said, "Did the doctors come in today? Did they talk about any change in your condition concerning you and the baby?"

Once again before I could answer him, he said with anticipation, "Has there been any change at all?"

I began to share with him everything the doctor had said. James suddenly got up from his chair and said, "I will be back."

I asked him, "Where are you going?"

At first, he would not look at me, and I said again, "James, where are you going?"

He looked back at me with tears in his eyes while his voice was cracking and said, "I am going to the nurses' station because I want to speak to the doctors myself."

"Please listen to what I am saying. There is nothing that we can do. This is what the doctors are telling me that was found in my bloodwork. The lupus is there. What do you expect the doctors to tell you differently from what they have told me?"

It's as if what I was saying to him was not what he wanted to hear. While he was gone, I lay staring into space because there was nothing I could do but feel helpless.

When James returned to my room, I asked him, "Were you able to speak to the doctor?"

He looked me in the eye and said, "Yes, I am so sorry for getting upset, and please forgive me. I just want my family to be okay."

We both began to hold each other's hands while trying to wipe our tears and pray. After we finished praying, James said he was going to leave and would bring Michelle up the next day, which would be Saturday morning, June 18. He kissed me goodnight, then he left.

I pulled my Bible out and attempted to read a Scripture that I had found, but I could not read. All I could get out was, "God please, please have mercy upon my soul."

It was 11:30 P.M., and I wanted to pray because all I had taken in my mind for the day was too much to bear. Though it was late, I felt like I needed to have one last talk with the Lord. I struggled to get out of bed and get down on my knees, but I managed to do so.

I said, "God, please let this baby be okay, and if for some reason I do not survive, please forgive me of all of my sins that I have committed in this life."

I was that sure that one of us would not be here the next day.

When I finished praying, I managed to struggle my way back into bed. The nurse came in with my nightly medications and a snack, which was a sandwich and some juice. After I ate, I sat up for a while just staring at nothing. After sitting for a while, I told myself I needed to try and get some rest. I slipped down into the covers while still lying on my back, when all of a sudden, I felt like my underclothes were damp. I knew I had not gone to the bathroom on myself, but I was too tired to check. Still lying there and wondering what was going on, I began to feel more dampness in my underclothes.

I said to myself, "God, what is going on with my body?"

The Lord spoke to me in that still small voice and said: "Call the nurse; your water has broken, and you are in labor."

May your unfailing love be my comfort, according
to your promise to your servant.
Let your compassion come to me that I may live, for your law is my delight.
(Psalm 119:76-77)

Chapter 8

PLEASE RESCUE ME

I was dumbfounded because I did not feel any pain, and I know when you are in labor and your water has broken, there should be some sort of pain, at least that is what I thought. I ignored the voice and what I felt, but then the voice of God spoke again, "Call the nurse. Your water has broken, and you are in labor."

I pushed the button for the nurse and she came into my room. She then looked at me with a smile and said, "Mrs. Forbes, may I help you?"

I felt silly and reluctant telling her that I thought my water had broken and I was in labor. Because if I were to tell her that the Lord had spoken to me and told me to call the nurse, I had a strange feeling she would not believe me. So, I simply told her, "I think that my water has broken."

She asked me if I had any pain, I told her, "No."

She said, "Mrs. Forbes, normally when you are in labor you will know it, and you will have some type of pain."

So, I said to her, "My underwear is damp. It feels like I just went to the bathroom on myself."

She said, "Well, let's take a look and see what may be going on."

As she examined me, she said, "I see some wetness, so what I am going to do is a simple test to see if you are really in labor. Give me a few minutes and I will be right back."

When she returned, she came back with another nurse and a kit in her hand. As she began to pull the covers back to do the examination, she began to explain what she would be doing. "Mrs. Forbes, I need you to lie completely still so that I can get a good reading from the test. What this kit will do is tell me if your water has broken. I am going to place this yellow strip on your abdomen, and if it turns blue within five minutes, your water has broken, and you are in labor."

Then she went on to say, "Like I said before, normally when you are in labor you will know it, and you will have some type of pain."

In my mind, I knew God must have heard my prayer and acted in an instant because I believed my water had surely broken.

After the five minutes had gone by, the nurse checked the strip she had placed on my abdomen. She looked at the other nurse and then she looked at me with a surprised look on her face and a smile with a little disbelief and said, "You are right—the strip is blue, and you are in labor. I need to contact the doctor right away, and I need to contact your husband. It is about 3:00A.M.; how soon do you think your husband can get here?"

I said to her, "He will get here in time." I was just that confident. There was one part of me that was so excited, and the other part was terrified.

As the nurse began to pull the blankets up over my body, she said, "Mrs. Forbes, please continue to lie still while I go and call the doctor. I will be right back."

The other nurse said, "Mrs. Forbes, if you start having severe pain, please push the call button, and one of us will come right away."

But as they left my room the strangest feeling came over me—it was a feeling almost like a premonition that I was going to die. I managed to get up out of bed and walk over to the chalkboard hanging on the wall. I began taking down the cards that I had received and reading the front of them while stacking them in a bundle in my hand. I had a bag that I began to put my personal items in, including my Bible. I felt like this was the end for me. My body was so calm, as though nothing was going wrong with me. In my mind, I knew God was carrying me in His arms, yet I felt taunted by the enemy in believing I was going to die.

I began walking back to the bed, and the nurse walked in looking startled and said, "Mrs. Forbes, what are you doing out of the bed? Do you realize the danger you could be putting you and your baby in?"

I looked at her with a stare wondering why she was so upset. I was not upset. It was as though my body was like a plane slowly descending. For some reason, I felt so free. Finally, two doctors (or maybe they were orderlies) came in with a stretcher, and one of them said, "We will be carrying you down to labor and delivery; the doctor and his team will be waiting."

Before they rolled me out, I asked the nurse, "Did you get in contact with my husband?"

The nurse said, "Mrs. Forbes, He is on his way, but we need to get you into labor and delivery now."

As I was being rolled down the hall, I had visions of my life as though the curtains of my life were being rolled back as I passed each room. Some parts of my life were wonderful, and some parts of my life were sad. I remember when I got to labor and delivery, there was a team of doctors there to greet me. They began to ask me how I was feeling, and all I could say was, "Okay."

They began to check my vitals, and I heard one doctor say, "We will have to move fast; her blood pressure is escalating, and we do not want the baby to go into distress."

One doctor asked the nurse, "Is her husband here yet? Because we need to move; the lupus is starting to flare up, and her vitals do not look good. We need to give her a high dose of Solu-Medrol (prednisone intravenously). This will get in to her system quickly to help control the lupus flare-up."

As I lay there while the doctors administered the Solu-Medrol by IV, I could hear the devil speaking to me in my mind. He said, "I have come to take you with me; you have nothing to live for."

I could feel my body going down into this deep, dark, cold hole. In my mind, I could hear myself trying to call out the name of Jesus, but the sound was so muffled. My eyes were open, and I looked around and felt as if a strong force tried to pull me down as I tried to pull up. I saw the phone on the wall, and I wanted to call my sister. Then I could hear the phone ringing several times, and the nurse came in to answer it.

She said, "Mrs. Forbes, if you can hear me, it is your sister on the phone; can you talk to her?"

I remember the nurse handing me the phone while holding it up to my ear. All I could hear was my sister praying for me and calling on the name of Jesus. She said, "Don't let the enemy take you—you have got to fight!"

As she prayed and spoke in the heavenly language of tongues, I could feel my body rising. The nurse took the phone from me and said, "We are taking you into the labor room now; the lupus has stabilized, and your husband and mom are here."

At this point I felt like the Lord heard my cry.

As they were wheeling me back, I had a chance to see my husband and my mom. They gave me an epidural injection in my spine to numb me. The doctors then performed an emergency Caesarian birth. They immediately handed the baby to the nurse, then to my husband. I was told that my mom also held her for a few minutes. I recall the nurses telling me that the baby came out smiling as my mom held her. The nurses said, "She is beautiful."

My husband said with tears in his eyes, "Not only is she beautiful, she is blessed, and Lillian and I are blessed that she is here."

Sheree came into this world on June 18, 1994, weighing six pounds and twelve ounces. They let me see her only for a few minutes then they took her to the Neonatal Intensive Care Unit (NICU) because she had hypoglycemia (low blood sugar). They also determined that her breathing was shallow. They put her on glucose intravenously for three days to raise her blood sugar. They eventually wheeled me back into the recovery room, where I stayed for several hours, still on the Solu-Medrol IV. The doctor told my husband, "Mr. Forbes, we need to watch Lillian closely because the lupus flared up so rapidly. This caused us to give her that strong dose of Solu-Medrol IV."

After several hours in recovery, they took me back to my room.

My eyes are ever on the Lord, for only he will release my feet from the snare.
Turn to me and be gracious to me, for I am lonely and afflicted.
Relieve the troubles of my heart and free me from my anguish.
Look on my affliction and my distress and take away all my sins.
(Psalm 25:15-18)

Chapter 9

LIFE UNDER CONSTRUCTION

I returned back to work February of 1995. Sheree was eight months old, and Michelle was now nine years old. I tried to adjust to working eight hours a day while dealing with the side effects from some of the medicines. It became overwhelming for me, and I found myself not being able to focus on my work. I began going to my job's health service unit three times a week, going through crying spells and small panic attacks. My supervisor then allowed me the time to go to the health service and rest for an hour every day if I needed to.

I felt like a new employee just starting a new job. Even though I had this job for eighteen years, I felt like I was in a strange place where I knew no one and no one knew me. One day while sitting at work I began to stare out the window, thinking back on how it had been ten months that I had not received a paycheck. I felt that I would probably have to work a few more weeks until I got one. I became depressed, but then as I was looking out the window, I saw a bird fly by, and I said to myself, *I am feeling fine, I feel free as that bird. I have overcome the worst of this disease. If God can take care of that bird, I knew He would continue to take care of me.*

I wanted to do my best to adjust to what was going on in my life, with my body, and with my family. I went to work every day, and I tried to keep a positive outlook. Even though I still was carrying weight in my stomach and my hair was still short, I wore makeup to try to cover my lesions, but I never could find the right color match for my skin. It felt as though no matter what kind I tried, the dark lesions still showed through the makeup. I tried to look past that and hoped everyone else would also.

I soon began to shy away from my coworkers and people I had known for years. When I would see them, I would pray to myself that they would keep walking and not stop to speak or ask me anything, especially asking me, "How are you feeling?" The pain was too deep inside of me, and it was still so fresh. I knew they knew me as someone different before I got sick, and I just didn't know how they felt toward me anymore. So many times you think you know your friends, and you think they will be there to see you through, but that was not my story or situation. I truly felt like some of the people I thought I was close to abandoned me. I am not sure if it was because of my illness and the fact that they could not handle it. Still, I needed them there for support. As time went on, I realized I had to rely on God and my family to help me cope. When I would see some of my friends and coworkers, it was as though I felt they could look right through me and see the pain I was experiencing. I still felt ugly inside and out.

I had a favorite skirt and sweater that I would wear at least two times a week. It was an aqua blue and green tropical print skirt. The sweater I wore with it was a sweater my mom had given me a long time ago, and it had the same print on it as the skirt. It was a heavy ivory sweater that had two thick appliqués of a tropical print sewn on each side of the sweater that made the sweater stand out. It was not a set, but I made it one. When I wore that outfit, it made me feel like I was on an island in a faraway land and that no one knew me.

People spoke to me every day asking me how I was feeling. They would say, "Welcome back to work."

They would stare at me in ways that made me feel so hurt. Though I could not read their minds, I could see their facial expressions as though they were surprised to see who they used to know looking so different. It was like being the new kid on the block. In my mixed-up mind, I knew I looked different, and I definitely felt different about myself. If I just tuned out the stares of the people I came into contact with whom I had known for years, I would be fine. It was like just meeting them for the first time and just not having too much to say. This is what made it easier for me to cope with people staring at me while I was at work. When the day ended and it was time to go home, my heart would skip an extra beat because I would say to myself, "Now I don't have to put on a show for the people on my job."

I was glad to get in the car where I could cry and let it all out. By the time I got home to my children, I was all cried out, and it was time to be mommy to them.

After the children were in bed, James and I talked about how we wanted to protect our girls from any hurt in all of this. We would often spend time talking with Michelle since she was a little older to make sure she knew how much she was loved despite what the family was going through. Yet, we began to notice Michelle starting to become quiet and not having much to say.

I suggested to James, "Maybe you need to talk with her while I am not around and hopefully she will open up."

James said, "No, we need to talk with her together so she can understand what you are feeling and what you are going through. I just feel that as her mother you need to let her know how much she is loved and that you are going to be okay. I feel this will give her more assurance coming from you and me together."

When I went upstairs to make sure Sheree was safely tucked in her crib, James went into Michelle's room and said to her, "Michelle, your mommy was sick, but she is getting better all the time, and she will not have to go back to the hospital or be away from you again. Mommy is going to come in and talk with you as soon as she puts Sheree in her crib."

Michelle said, "Daddy, I miss Mommy when she is not here, and I don't want her to keep leaving me and Sheree."

As I was entering Michelle's room, I heard her say those words to James, and I just felt like my heart would break in two. I went directly to her and sat on the bed, holding her in my arms, and I said to her, "Michelle, Mommy loves you and Sheree so much, and it breaks my heart every time I have to be away from you. I know you miss me, and I miss you too, but mommy needs to get better, and that is why she has to keep going away to the hospital."

Immediately I began to cry as I held her so tightly in my arms and close to my heart. As I gently laid her back down on her pillow, I wiped her tears away along with mine. Kissing her forehead, I smiled at her with more love then a mother could ever give.

James looked into Michelle's big brown eyes and said, "Baby girl, I miss her when she is not here too, and I want her to get better so she can always be with us." James then kissed her on her forehead too and told her, "God loves you and so do we."

Once we went to sleep, I often got up and would sneak downstairs to eat ice cream and yogurt. When I came back to bed, James would sometimes ask, "Lil, where were you?"

"I was checking on the children."

I knew that I was not telling the truth, but in my mind, I did not care because eating ice cream and yogurt and sneaking to do it, made me feel like I was in control. I was going to do just what I wanted to do. Even if I was in control just for that short span of time, it brought me comfort at the end of the day. I was sick and tired of eating bland food in order to keep my blood sugar stable.

The next morning when I got up, I went through the routine of getting my children together and then getting myself together. I could never find anything to wear, and I was tired of wearing the maternity clothes to work. My stomach was going down slowly since they had lowered the dose of my prednisone, but I could not understand why my weight was still 165 pounds. I had never weighed that much before in my life. I was forty pounds over my normal weight. As time went on and I was still working, trying to keep it together, I began to have severe pains in the bottom of my stomach. I called my doctor, and he had me to schedule an appointment for a sonogram. After the sonogram, I received a phone call from my doctor's office and the nurse said, "Mrs. Forbes, it appears that you have a hernia that has developed in the stomach wall. The doctor would like to schedule a date for surgery to repair the hernia, so that you will not continue to be in pain."

I knew I needed to have this done because the pain was unbearable at times, and it was hard to eat anything and keep it down. I also knew I had to talk with my supervisor again, which was something I did not want to do. I felt like I had just returned to work, and I already needed to leave again. The next day, I went to work and asked my supervisor if I could meet with her. We met in her office, and I began to tell her, "I am so sorry but I have to take off again and I know I do not have any leave. I'm afraid of losing my job because I've been away so long."

My supervisor calmly said, "Mrs. Forbes, it's okay. I know you are under a lot of stress, and I know you are still dealing with a lot. Just let me know when you will be out so we can handle the necessary paperwork."

As I got up from my chair, I looked at her with tears in my eyes and all I could say was, "Thank you for being so understanding. I am really sorry."

She said, "It is not your fault. We will take care of it."

I felt like I was in the storm once again with no chance of getting out. I felt like I kept going through the same revolving door that always brought me back to the same desolate place in my life. I had some bloodwork done before the hernia surgery, and they said my numbers looked good, including my blood sugar. So we scheduled the surgery for the middle of July of 1995 at Georgetown University Hospital. They repaired the hernia, and once again I was out of work for a period of ten days. When I returned to work, I tried to act as though my life was fine.

When I came home from work, I resumed my normal motherly routine, and at night I was still sneaking downstairs, eating the ice cream and yogurt. I slipped backward, day by day, but I tried to hide it from my family. I had thoughts of not wanting to deal with any of this anymore. Still, I always thought about my children and how I wanted to be there for them.

I had a follow-up appointment with my doctor in September, and I had bloodwork done. I received a phone call at home from the doctor's office and the nurse said, "Mrs. Forbes, your bloodwork came back, and the doctor is concerned about your results. He would like for you to call him so he can talk with you directly."

I said, "Okay" and hung up. At that moment, all I could think was, *Here I go again. Is this the end for me?*

I told James what the doctor said, and he said, "We have been down this road before, so we will just hear what he says and take it from there."

I looked at him and immediately became upset with him. I was upset because this was my life and my body, and even though he has been with me, I told James, "You have no idea what goes on in my mind and my body on a daily basis. You only know what I choose to share."

But I could not tell him how I truly felt because I knew he was doing his best to try and be my comfort through all of this.

The next day, I called the doctor to discuss the results and he said, "Mrs. Forbes I am troubled with your bloodwork. Your protein in your urine has elevated and your sugar is extremely high. I need to ask you: are you watching what you eat and are you staying away from foods that are high in sugar?"

I didn't exactly tell the doctor what I should have told him while I was there; I told him that I was watching what I was eating.

He then said, "We are going to check your bloodwork in another week to see if anything has changed, but until then, please stick to your diet."

I said, "Okay" and we left. As time began to pass, I was not sticking to my diet like I should have. There were things I wanted to eat, and I tried to do it in moderation—at least I thought I was. There were nights when I was still sneaking my ice cream and the TCB Yogurt, which was high in sugar. Later during the week, I had bloodwork done and after the bloodwork I went to spend time with my mom. I was not feeling that great, but I wanted to get out of the house. My mom came to pick up me and my children. We spent the day and half of the evening with her. James was going to come and pick us up after he got home from work. I remember as I was sitting at my mom's, I said to her, "Mom I need to lie down. I don't feel too well, and my eyes feel funny as though they have sand or grit in them."

My mom said, "You go and lie across the bed until James comes, and I will watch the children."

As soon as I lay down, a half hour passed, and the phone rang. It was James, and he said "I am coming to get you now! The doctor called and left a message on the phone and said to bring you back to the hospital right away. Your blood sugar is 860, and that is stroke range. You have to come back to the hospital today."

James came to pick me up, and we took the children to the babysitter next door.

I was frozen with silence; I did not know what to say. When we got to the hospital and I was checked into my room, my doctor came in to see me. I had a look of shame on my face. I then held my head down and said, "I kind of went off my diet, and I'm sorry."

"Mrs. Forbes, do you realize how serious this is? We are talking about your life! You have to do what you are told to do in order to get better. You could have had a stroke at any time. I want you to stay here in this hospital until we can bring your sugar down to a level that we are comfortable with."

Again, all I could think about was my children and what I had just talked to Michelle about. I told her that I would not be away from them again. I lay there in the bed with a blank look on my face. It was as though someone just stuck a knife in my heart, and I was bleeding a slow death.

The doctor called the nurse into my room, and he was giving her instructions on what medications to give me in order to bring my sugar level down. After the doctor finished talking to the nurse he said, "Mrs. Forbes I will be back in the morning to check on you, but the nurse has some instructions that she will be going over with you when she comes back."

They both left the room, and I was relieved and embarrassed because this was something that I did to myself and did not consider the consequences it would create for my family. I looked at James and said, "James, I was sneaking downstairs at night while you were sleeping eating ice cream and some other things."

James looked at me with disappointment in his eyes and said, "You know better. How you are going to get better if you keep doing things the doctors tell you not to do? You have got to stop it! I am doing my best to help you. I want you to get better, but it's like you are not trying to get better. Have you gone back to being depressed? If so, tell me, so we can get you some help. I want this family together and I want you well. I know you want that too. So please, let's try to get through this together."

I said, "James I am sorry, but I am mentally and physically tired. I will try to do better, and yes, I find myself slipping back into depression."

James said, "Once this episode is over ,we will look into getting you some help."

"I do not want any help. I am not crazy. I just want to be left alone."

He then said, "I am not going to leave you alone because I love you and you need someone to talk to besides me and one way or another we are going to do this. The first thing I am going to do is call your job so I can talk with your supervisor."

I begged him to please not say anything about me not doing what I was supposed to do, because that is what brought me back to the hospital. I did not want my supervisor or my family to know. He assured me that he would not do that to me, but made me promise him that I would stop this nonsense of not listening to the doctor. I said that I would because I felt bad for what I had done.

The next day James called my job and talked with my supervisor. I stayed in the hospital for a week on a strict diet. They increased my insulin and my prednisone again to help with the protein. I did not want them to increase the prednisone because it messed with my mind so much and added to my depression. Once my sugar was stable and the protein had decreased in my urine, I was released to go home.

I returned to work in the middle of September. I went back to my lifestyle as I knew it. I was still taking the medications and trying to follow my diet daily. It was so hard for me to not sneak downstairs at night, but I had to realize if I wanted to get better, I had to do what the doctors said.

My mom called me one evening and said, "Look, I know you are tired and you want to get well, but you have to listen to what the doctors are telling you, please. James told me what happened and why you are there, James also said he would not tell me but he felt that I needed to know what was really going on."

After hearing the concern in my mother's voice over the phone, I told my mother that I would, but I started crying and said to her, "But Mom, I am tired, and it's so hard for me."

She said she loved me and told me to try to get some rest. Once I got off the phone, James and I put the children to bed and, then I tried to get some rest. I could not sleep right away because I had to ask James about what my mom said. So, I asked him, "Why did you tell my mom when you said you would not?"

He said, "Because I love you, and I want you here with me and our children."

I quietly said, "I understand," and I lay down to rest. I tried to do more with my family and my children as the months went by.

One day, I looked in the mirror and noticed that my hair seemed to be growing back but also getting thinner in other areas. I also noticed swelling again around my ankles. They had become tight, and my urine looked darker again. I became worried once again.

Heal me, Lord and I will be healed; save me and
I will be saved, for you are the one I praise.
(Jeremiah 17:14)

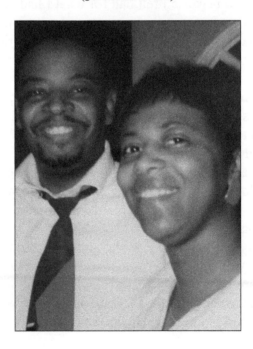

Chapter 10

MY BODY STILL FEELS BROKEN

I had an appointment to see my doctor on November 6, and I wanted to hear some good news for once. I was tired of getting bad reports about my health each time I saw my doctor. I hoped for good news because my birthday was coming up right after the Thanksgiving holiday. I went to see my doctor, and after he completed his examination he said, "Mrs. Forbes, I notice you have swelling around your ankles again, and there is some discoloration in your skin. I am going to order some bloodwork, and I would like to do a biopsy of your kidneys."

After hearing the news, the doctor just gave me, my thought of enjoying the Thanksgiving holiday and my birthday suddenly meant nothing. I was in no mood to celebrate anything.

The doctor went on to say, "The nurse will call you and set up the appointment for the biopsy. It will only be an overnight stay in the hospital. If you like, we can schedule it for a weekend; that way you won't have to take leave from work. I know that has been a concern of yours. Once we have the results, I will call you. In the meantime, try to stay off your feet as much as possible and get some rest."

There was no conversation between James and me in the car the entire ride home. Our silence finally broke when he asked me, "How do you feel?"

I looked at him and said, "I am scared, and I don't want to talk about it."

I went to work the next day as though the doctor had not told me anything. I came home and did my same routine, but still there was little conversation between James and me. One afternoon while I was at work, I decided to go outside for lunch. I called James and asked him if he would walk outside with me for lunch. As we walked, I started saying a few words here and there because I did not want anyone to think there was anything wrong between us.

I said to him, "James, I am really scared, and I don't know what to do."

I held back tears because I was still at work.

James said, "I know you are afraid, and I am too, but we have to trust God. And I want you to know that I am going to be here for you along with your family. I know it seems like an answer you don't want to hear, but I just don't have any more answers to give you. And if it helps, I love you very much."

After I came back to my desk and checked my phone, there was a message from my doctor. I called my doctor back, and the nurse asked if we could come to the office tomorrow because my doctor wanted to talk with us.

The next day, James and I went to see my doctor. He told us to come in and have a seat. "Mrs. Forbes, the lupus is flaring up again, raising its ugly head, causing more protein to spill from the kidneys. We have to try to attack this from a different angle because your urine is getting a little darker. The creatinine levels are a little higher, more than what we want to see."

All I could do was ask him, "How are you going to treat this? What will you be doing?"

James said, "Doctor I need you to really explain to us what is going on here. I thought Lillian was getting better. She goes to work every day, she has some swelling and fatigue, and she is still going to the bathroom. It is not as much as you would like, but she is going."

"Mr. Forbes, the protein can only be seen in the bloodwork, and I am certain she notices the darkness of her urine. We will do more bloodwork and see how much damage is being done to her kidneys. The kidneys are in danger of failing because of the lupus. So, we would like to start your wife on cyclophosphamide, which is a type of chemo. Another term for this chemo is Cytoxan."

James immediately said, "What is that?"

Before the doctor could answer James, I just blurted out, "What side effects are these treatments going to have? Am I going to feel sicker than I am already feeling?"

He said, "Mrs. Forbes, I can see the concerned look in your eyes, and I am going to be honest with you as much as I can. The side effects can be nausea, loss of appetite, mouth sores, hair loss, black stool, and extreme fatigue. Most of these side effects, you have already experienced from the lupus, so I'm hoping you will adjust to the treatments."

Then the doctor went on to answer James: "Mr. Forbes, this is a drug given by infusion intravenously to treat different forms of cancer and certain cases of lupus nephritis. Your wife's autoimmune disease, which is the systemic lupus erythematosus (SLE), has caused severe scarring to her kidneys, which is causing the kidney failure. The treatments will be done here at Georgetown for a period of two years. You will have to start this treatment soon. This will be handled as an outpatient treatment, and you will be reporting to the oncology unit when you arrive. You will receive all the paper work from my nurse, and she will give you information on this type of chemo."

As the doctor walked out of his office, the nurse came in. She began to explain to me and my husband what to expect and what would cause them to not give me the treatment on a particular day. She proceeded to say, "If you have a cold or a fever, or if your blood pressure is elevated, you will not receive your treatment. You will be admitted the last Friday of every third month to receive your treatments. We will be giving you the drug by infusion from 9:00 in the morning until 5:30 in the evening. You will have to complete eight to ten cycles of the cyclophosphamide pulses of this chemo in order for us to see some positive results. You will complete your last cycle of the drug in September of 1997."

The doctor then walked back in the office and said, "We would like to start you on the treatment the third Friday in December of 1995, and then the last Friday of every third month, so we can be on a schedule as planned. Mrs. Forbes, I know this is an awful lot for you to take in, but we have to do this in order to try and save your kidneys."

This time I sat there and I cried out loud as long as someone would listen to me. I wanted them to see and feel my pain. I could not express my hurt and disappointment with words, so all I could do was just cry. No one bothered me for a moment, and they let me cry and get it all out. The nurse brought me some water and tissues and gave me a hug.

James said to the doctor, "Is this going to help her kidneys, and in what way?"

The doctor said, "Mr. Forbes, the chemo will actually slow down the spreading of the lupus attacking your wife's body, especially her kidneys. And we hope and pray that this will put the lupus in remission. I cannot tell you this is a cure because it is not, but it will slow the progression of the disease."

James said, "Lillian, I know this is a lot and I don't know what to say to you to make things better, but let's just go home and pray about this."

So, we got up, and James shook the doctor's hand and the nurse rubbed my back while the doctor said, "Mrs. Forbes please get some rest and try not to upset yourself any more then you have. We will get a grip on this ugly disease."

As James and I walked to the car, the weather outside was cold, and so was my heart. I told him, "I do not want to go home right now. Can you please call the babysitter and ask her if we could be a little late getting the children?"

We walked around for a little while until we found a bench to sit on near a park. I looked up into the sky, looking at the clouds and their different shades of gray from the cold.

I said to James, "The clouds look light as a feather, like they do not have a care in the world. It looks as though they don't have anything weighing them down. I wish I could go up there."

James said, "Please don't talk like that. I want you to fight, and I want you to fight to win."

But I told him, "I just don't have any more fight left in me," and my eyes began to swell with tears.

I said, "I have to tell my mom and I have to let my supervisor know that I will be at Georgetown getting this chemo. Does this mean that I am really going to die? When people get chemo, doesn't that mean that there is no more they can do for them?"

James said, "I don't think so. You heard the doctor say that he is hoping this would slow the progression down of the lupus, and that is what we have to pray for."

As we got up from the bench and began to walk to our car, I said to James, "I do not want to tell Michelle. Just let me deal with this my way because I am having a hard time trying to process this."

Blessed is the one who perseveres under trial because,
having stood the test, that
person will receive the crown of life that the Lord has
promised to those who love him.
(James 1:12)

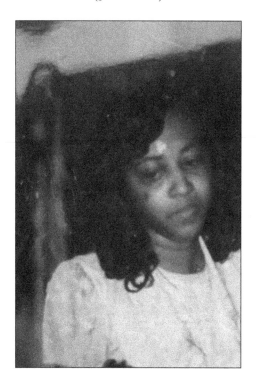

Chapter 11

LIVING AND NOT KNOWING

W hen I returned to work the following week, I once again had a meeting with my supervisor and she approved my LWOP for the treatments. I explained to her all of the details of what my doctor told me. Suddenly, I stopped in the middle of my conversation, and said, "Do you think I will lose my job? I do not have any money saved up, and my husband is working part time at another job. Things are hard."

My supervisor said, "Mrs. Forbes, let's not talk about that right now. We will discuss that at a later date. Right now, you have so much more to be concerned with like your children and your health. We will let tomorrow take care of itself for right now."

I did not want to hear that because I had no money, and I was disgusted with life and everything in it. After I went home from work that evening, James and I decided to call my mom. We told her we wanted to have a family meeting with everyone.

I discussed the issue with my mom and my family, and they were sympathetic to all that I was going through. I felt like they knew they had to be in order to help me to get through this.

I could see the concern on my mom's face and on my brothers' and sisters' faces as well. There was nothing I could do but look away. I did not want them to see me crying.

As James and I left to come back home, I was completely silent. He was talking to the girls and making little jokes while driving along. All I could think about was Christmas and how I wanted to be well to enjoy that special time with my children. I did not want to feel sick and be in bed feeling bad and in terrible pain. To me, Christmas is a time for love, a time for family, and a special time to remember Jesus. It was hard to even put those thoughts in my mind or feel them in my heart.

I started my treatments in December of 1995. I had convinced myself to try my best to have a positive attitude through all of this because I wanted my children to have a wonderful Christmas, and I wanted it to be the best ever. On the day of the treatments, my husband would take me to Georgetown on Friday morning, and I would go through the routine of having my temperature taken and my blood drawn. After the doctors saw that my temperature was fine, and my bloodwork was good, they began the infusion treatments of the chemo. I lay in the bed all day receiving the treatment. They would bring me a sandwich and a small cup of juice because I was told I could not have a lot of liquids while the treatment was being administered.

James would come to the hospital at exactly 5:30 P.M. to pick me up and bring me home. When I got home, I would be very tired after the treatments but I knew I had to continue down this road. The doctor had given me a prescription for a particular type of medicine that I was supposed to drink in the evening before I went to bed after each treatment. This medicine was to coat my bladder and my liver from the strong chemo that I was being given. I remember drinking it and spitting it out because the taste was so nasty.

As time went on I continued the treatments, I made myself adjust to the taste of the medicine. The chemo was strong, and there were days that it affected my breathing. I remember my husband taking me to the local hospital emergency room because I felt like something was cutting off my windpipe. I actually felt like someone was holding a pillow over my nose and mouth trying to suffocate me. Once we got to the hospital and in the emergency room, they ran tests after my husband gave them a history of my illness. They immediately did a test to see the oxygen level in my blood.

After so many hours of lying in the emergency room waiting on the results, the doctor came into the room and said, "Mrs. Forbes, we have the results back, and what has happened is the oxygen level in your blood has decreased, which is why you feel as though something is cutting off your air. This is one of the side effects from taking the chemo. We are going to give you a prescription, and we want you to follow up with your doctor."

In the meantime, they gave me something to make me feel better along with an inhaler for the shortness of breath. I continued to work and try my best to adapt to the changes that I was still going through. My children were everything to me, and my focus was making sure that I could shelter them from all of this, but sometimes that was impossible. There were times when I would snap at my children and my husband. Michelle was now ten going on eleven, and there were things she wanted to do with her mother, but I was too tired to do them. My doctor called me before my next treatment was due to tell me that my blood count was low and that they needed to give me at least two blood transfusions in order to continue the treatments. I was scared because I knew receiving blood from someone else could be dangerous. I expressed that to my doctor, and he said, "Please know we have taken every precaution to make sure that we give you your correct blood type, and this blood has been checked for any kind of contamination."

I said to him, "I am going to trust you even though I am scared. I have come to the end of my rope, and I am tired so I am going to trust that through all of these treatments, I will get better."

I received the two blood transfusions and continued the treatments. I had to receive a total of five transfusions during the course of my chemo treatments. My hair continued to get thinner as I was going through the chemo, and my weight appeared to stay the same. As I looked at myself, still I was so unhappy with my outer appearance until it affected everything about me that my heart was supposed to feel after giving birth. I never had a moment of enjoying that special bonding time after giving birth to Sheree. I was supposed to be enjoying life to its fullest. All that I thought was good was all gone to me. I imagined that it felt like every time I kept going to the well for fresh clean water, the well was always full of dirty unclean water. I was thirsty for something new; I was thirsty for fresh water to drink in my life. Yet, the well began to run dry for me when I would go to find peace, whether it was in prayer or trying to talk to my mom and my husband. Nothing anyone said was making sense to me. They kept telling me that in time things would get better and that God heard my prayers. To me, no one understood and no one heard me when I cried for help. It was like cries in the dark in my mind. I needed a breakthrough, and I needed it now.

I felt like things were closing in on me faster then I wanted them to. I felt like the oxygen that was low in my blood was suffocating me completely as a person. I couldn't breathe. I started to become empty on the inside. Every time I turned around, I was either in the doctor's office for bad news or in the hospital because something else had been discovered. I started to wonder if there would ever be a rainbow in the sky for me to see.

I was walking along this dark path while looking up into a dark sky. It was then that I believe the Lord heard my cry because on September 5, 1997, I was able to stop my chemo treatments. My doctor ran more blood tests after the treatments and called me to set up an appointment to come into his office. James and I met with the doctor on September 9, 1997 and he said to us, "Mrs. Forbes, I have some great news to tell you and your husband. The chemo treatments that you were given has slowed the lupus down, and I think it is safe to say that your lupus has gone into remission. Since the lupus appears to be in remission, we will stop the prednisone completely for now."

I heard what the doctor said as I watched James sitting with tears in his eyes as a sign of relief. My mind had begun to travel back to that dreadful day as I sat in the doctor's office and heard I had this "chronic disease called lupus." I was so happy to hear the news, but it didn't show on my face.

The doctor must have thought I had lost my mind because he said, "Mrs. Forbes, did you hear the good news I just gave you and your husband?"

I said, "Yes I heard everything you said, but are you sure that I am in remission? I just cannot take any more disappointments in my life; I want to be well completely so I can enjoy my life and raise my children."

The doctor said, "You now have a chance to do this. Please look at this as a time to take in all of the wonderful things about life that you have missed, especially time you have wanted to spend with your children."

He reminded me that even though my body was in remission, my immune system was still compromised. I got up from my chair and told the doctor, "Thank you for all that you have done to help me."

When James and I left the doctor's office, James said, "Let's go have lunch and celebrate this blessing."

I said okay, even though I was not in a mood to celebrate; I still felt like this was just a temporary fix to a problem that was never going away. I just didn't want to get my hopes up to be let down with more disappointments. I began to cry as we were driving along. I just could not hold it in any longer. It was such good news to hear, but the reminder of all that I had gone through kept overshadowing the good news I had just received.

After we had lunch, I came home and called my mom to tell her. She began to thank God for His blessing in hearing the prayers of our family. Our wedding anniversary was coming up soon, so we decided after all that we had been through, we would take time and go away.

On September 17, 1997, James and I celebrated our fifteenth wedding anniversary. We knew we wanted our children with us wherever we went, so we decided just to go somewhere local and stay at a nice hotel. We ended up going to Baltimore and staying at The Harbor. That way we could enjoy some sightseeing and spend time with James' family.

We had a wonderful time and talked about our plans for wanting to move out of our townhouse into a single-family home. We did not have a lot of money saved because of my medications and hospital bills. Even though I had health insurance and qualified for Medicare because of my end-stage renal failure, everything was still not covered. We talked about so many things that we wanted to do. We made it a priority to talk with a financial counselor about helping us in order to get on the right path to buying a new home. That day after hearing the good news, it was as though we got a new lease on life. Everything felt so beautiful—every moment that was captured with everything we did and said from that moment on meant so much to each of us. My family was together, and I was a mother and a wife again.

Jesus said "This sickness will not end in death.
No, it is for God's glory so that God's Son may be glorified through it."
John 11:4

Chapter 12

MY FANTASY WORLD

A year had gone by since chemotherapy, and I was still working and trying to capture all the time of my life that I felt I had lost. We were still trying to move, hoping God would bless us with a bigger house to raise our children. With the blessing of hearing the good news about the lupus, we felt like we wanted to have a home and not just a house. I began to feel differently about myself as I started to see small changes taking place in my body and appearance. Though the lesions were still on my face and over my body, I took in a deep breath within my spirit, and I began to breathe.

On January 30, 1999, I had a doctor's appointment with my rheumatologist. He discussed some of the bloodwork and urine test results he had received with me. The doctor told me my creatinine level in my blood was beginning to elevate again, which showed that my kidneys were still not properly functioning.

The doctor said, "Mrs. Forbes, we would like to rebiopsy the kidney." He also said that once they got the results back, they would like to try a new treatment. The doctor said, "We want to do everything we can in order to preserve your kidneys. You are young, and we want to see you enjoying your life."

In February of 1999, I had the biopsy done, and the doctor called to tell me there was a lot of scarring still in the kidney from the lupus. The doctor also said, "There are about twenty little lesions lying on your abdomen, and we feel they are there from the lupus. They are too small for us to biopsy, so we are going to leave them alone. If your stomach starts to really hurt, let us know, and we will study that further to see what can be done."

He then said, "This normally appears as lesions from the lupus, and that is another reason why your stomach looks as though it not going down, but in time it will. What we would like to do is increase your blood pressure medicines to see if that will take less strain off the kidney and keep your blood pressure low."

Fridays were the day of the week when most of my appointments were scheduled. I thought that was great for me because whatever devastating news I would receive, it gave me time over the weekend to process it before returning to work. I had an appointment on May 27, 1999, and the doctor was pleased with my progress.

He said, "Increasing the blood pressure medicine has taken some strain off of the kidneys."

I was no longer on the prednisone, so he asked me, "How do you feel?"

I told him, "I feel well overall, but I am still experiencing a lot of fatigue."

I would dare not tell him how I felt about this whole situation. I felt like I had been cheated out of having a happy life, I felt like a mother who was abandoning her children even though I was there with them most of the time. I felt like the doctors and God owed me an explanation and a new life. As crazy as it sounds, somebody needed to give me back the life that was stolen from me with this ugly, ugly disease. But I knew I could not share that with my doctor for the fear of thinking he would want to prescribe some type of antidepressant medication. I felt like another medication would be the last thing I would need.

I saw my doctor again on July 20, 1999, and he was still pleased with my progress. One day, while we were at home, James said, "We are still going to move. I don't know how, but I believe it's going to happen, and I want you to believe it too. I want you to look at me when I tell you that my heart hurts like yours does. It tears me up inside to see you go through all of this. I sometimes cry at night while you and the girls are asleep. I asked the Lord to please bring some sunshine into our lives, to please make a way financially so that we can move into a larger home for our family."

I looked back at him and said, "James, I want to have faith and be as strong as you are, but it is so hard for me. I feel like I am in a bad dream and cannot wake up."

He then said, "Please hold on. Hold on to me and onto God. I believe He is going to see us through."

I said to him, "Because you have asked me to, I will try harder."

We were going into a new year and still going through the same daily routine of doctor visits and bloodwork.

Every two months, I went to the doctor, and during my June appointment, my doctor said, "Mrs. Forbes, your kidney function is stable, and your creatinine is at a good level. Your blood pressure is well controlled by the medications. Continue to do what you are doing, and we will continue to follow up with you."

I saw my doctor again on August 18, 1999, and continued to receive a good report overall with my health. The lupus was still in remission, and the kidney was still stable.

On October 16, 1999, the Lord found favor with James and me, and we were blessed with our new home. We were so happy and thankful that God heard our prayers. My attitude about my life and myself had shifted to positive again. I was looking forward to decorating our new home and filling it with love and newness of life. I told myself I wanted to leave behind a lot of memories from my other home. I felt this was a new beginning, even though I knew I could never forget everything that I experienced while living in my other home. The scars were on my body, and the pain was still in my heart.

The main thing was my children were happy, and everyone in our family was happy for us. From the time the doctor told me in September that the lupus was in remission, I was trying to do as much in my life as possible that was positive because I never knew when I would fall down again.

I returned to church on a regular basis and became more involved again. I was a part of the laity in my church, and it felt good to go back and be a part of something that was always special to me. I knew I had a lot to give God thanks for, even though some areas in my spiritual walk was still weak because of the pain I carried with me.

Create in me a pure heart, O God, and renew a steadfast spirit within me.
Do not cast me from your presence or take your Holy Spirit from me.
Restore to me the joy of your salvation and grant me a willing spirit, to sustain me.
(Psalm 51:10-12)

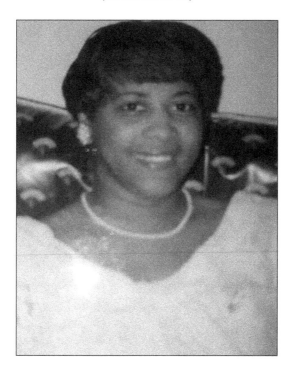

Chapter 13

TRYING TO COPE

B y February 2, 2000, I was still going to the doctor, repeating the same test, but I was thankful because things still looked good for me.

In April of 2000, my doctor said, "Mrs. Forbes, you are doing well," and he still felt my lupus was under control."

I was still so happy to hear the great news that the doctor shared with me. My appointments were starting to spread out over time because my lupus had quieted down.

I told James, "This all started in 1994, and I am still going to the doctor and doing monthly bloodwork and a urine test after all these years. It just seems so unreal to me. Six years and I am still seeing the same doctors at the same hospital."

All my husband could say was, "I don't understand it, but I am sure it's all in God's plan because you are still here with us."

That made me feel good, and it helped inspire me to keep looking at the positive side of this whole situation. My husband and I planned trips with our kids and the rest of our family. We enjoyed life and had a wonderful time. I watched my children grow right before my eyes. I still felt that I had missed out on so much with them through the years, and I said to myself that I wanted to make every moment count with both of them. I was doing so much in my life now, and being busy helped me not to dwell on what I was going through or the pain that no one but God will ever understand.

The seasons changed, and I began to notice swelling in my ankles, and my skin lesions had begun to spread more over different areas of my body. I hoped nothing was wrong again. I also had a strange taste in my mouth, as though I had been eating something that was made of metal. I told James that I kept getting this strange taste in my mouth.

James said, "Metal? What are you talking about?"

I told him, "That is what my mouth tastes like. It feels as though someone just fed me a box of nails. The taste is terrible, and it makes my food taste the same way."

He then asked me, "Have you noticed anything with your urine like a change in color or a decrease?"

"Not really. I know that I have a doctor's appointment this week, so if anything is wrong they can catch it."

Later that week, when I got to the doctor's office, the doctor said, "How are you feeling?"

I looked at James and hesitated to answer because I knew I had not been completely honest with the doctors before. I told the doctor, "I have started to experience different things in my body: I'm experiencing a metal taste in my mouth and some numbness and tingling around my mouth and in my fingertips and hands."

The doctor said, "We are going to start you on a baby aspirin daily, and we have ordered another lupus workup because some of your results from your bloodwork have us concerned again. Once all the tests are back, I will call you and discuss them with you. Mrs. Forbes, I can see the worry in your eyes, but I want you to stay calm until I have the entire battery of tests back."

My only reaction to him was "Is this lupus trying to raise its ugly head again in my life?"

The doctor said, "I don't know, but I will contact you as soon as I have the results back."

A week went by, and I began to feel scared and worried. I found myself slowly drifting back into a shell.

About a week later, the results of the tests I had taken came back that the doctor had ordered at the beginning of August. My doctor called and said, "We think the lupus is trying to flare up again. What we would like to do is put you on a drug called CellCept."

I asked him, "What type of drug is this?"

"It is a pill form similar to the chemo that you had taken. We are hoping it will help to keep your lupus in remission. This has fewer side effects than the Cytoxan. It is used to prevent organ rejection in transplant patients and is sometimes used for treatment in certain autoimmune diseases such as lupus. We will also put you back on the prednisone, but it will be a low dose. Our goal is to try to do everything we can to save your kidneys."

I simply said, "Okay. When do I start?"

I started taking the CellCept at the end of August 2000. I started taking the medication twice a day, once in the morning and once in the evening. I began to notice myself having mood swings, I was unable to sleep at night, and I was experiencing some dizziness. Though the doctor said the side effects were not that bad, the drug began to play with my mind. By this time in my life, I began again to sink back into a low point of depression. I found myself not engaging in conversations with my coworkers or even with my family. James would try to talk to me, but my answers to him were only a yes or a no. I pushed myself to become available just enough to care for my children. It almost felt like I was playing house with my family. I cooked for them, washed clothes, cleaned the house, spent time with my children, and of course I still had to go to work.

When people would see me, whether at work or at church, I would smile as though everything was great. I talked about how I was coping with my illness and how James and I tried to take it one day at a time, working it out together. I never spoke of the many nights I sat up crying, looking at myself, and saying I hated myself and hated life. I felt as though I had been dealt a rotten hand of cards, and it was totally unfair. I wished this had happened to someone else and not me. I would even search on the computer to see if the doctors had missed anything that might be a cure for me. But I could never find anything.

The doctors were still monitoring my urine output and still taking bloodwork. My body and my mind tried to adjust to the CellCept as I continued to go on with my life. The CellCept began to cause so many side effects until the doctor took me off of it in February 2001. I found myself coming home in the evenings and going directly to my bedroom. I would sit on the bed and twirl my hair and stare at the wall. I felt if I found a focal point where I could fix my eyes on something; it would help me not to think so much about what was happening around me.

James would call out to me from downstairs to ask me if I was okay. I would say, "Yes, I am fine, and I will be right down."

I would take an ink pen and mark the spot on the wall so when I came back, I would know where I was sitting and where I was looking. Believe it or not, that was therapy for me.

After I cooked for my family, I would return back upstairs and just sit until it was time to put the kids to bed. James would clean up the kitchen and then would come upstairs to ask me what was wrong. I would answer him by saying, "Nothing is wrong. Everything is wonderful. Can't you tell?"

He would look at me with hurt in his eyes because he could see I hadn't accepted that this was happening again as I was trying my best to cope.

Therefore we do not lose heart. Though outwardly we are wasting away,
yet inwardly we are being renewed day by day. For our light and momentary
troubles are achieving for us an eternal glory that far outweighs them all.
(Second Corinthians 4:16-17)

Chapter 14

LOSING MY MIND

In 2001, I was still going to doctor appointments, completing the same tests with the same doctors. The holidays would come and go along with the birthdays, but I always made sure that my children would have a wonderful Christmas and special birthdays.

When I saw my doctor again, I told him I was having digestive issues and noticed that my stools were darker. He was concerned that I might have gastro-intestinal (GI) bleeding. I had to have a stool test done to rule out any type of bleeding. When I got my results back, I said, "Thank God it's okay."

This seemed to be the only other time that anything looked good in my favor.

The continuing effects of illness had gotten old to me by now, and I was still just going through the motions of trying to be happy. I continued to get more rashes on my body and more skin lesions. My doctor said, "The skin lesions appear to be what's known as discoid lupus." He gave me some cream and wanted me to try that for a while, but he also said, "I suggest you see a dermatologist for the rash and the lesions."

So, I made an appointment to see the dermatologist, and she gave me a topical cream for my face, arms, legs, and back.

Over time, the cream helped, but it never took away the scars. I continually changed makeup to cover up my scars. One evening when I came home from work, James said, "I'm going to take the kids out to get a bite to eat so you can have some time to yourself. Do you want me to bring you something back?"

I told him I did not want anything and that I would find something to eat in the house. I was so relieved when they left because I could go upstairs and have a crying pity party by myself. When they returned, James asked me, "Lil, have you gotten some rest?"

Of course, I lied and said, "Yes."

After the children were asleep, James said, "I'm going to buy you some new pillows and a new bedspread to brighten this room because you spend so much time in here and the colors are so dark."

Little did he know that the bedroom was a reflection of my life to me.

James bought me some new fluffy down pillows, which were soft to sleep on, and he also purchased a new bedspread and comforter. It was pretty in color—green and yellow, which made the room look bright.

My doctors were still monitoring me because of my flare-up with the lupus. They were still checking my creatinine levels, which slowly rose. I felt I was slowly being tortured for a crime I did not commit. I felt as though I was held hostage in a prison that had no name. I found myself slowly sinking lower and lower as time went on.

One evening, I came up to my bedroom, and as I lay down, I noticed something kept sticking in my head from the pillow. I then took the pillowcase off and feathers began to poke through the pillow. I told James that we had to get new pillows because the feathers kept sticking out of them. I continued to sleep on them anyway.

This particular evening, James decided to take the children out again to give me a break, so I went upstairs and my mind went right to the pillow. I took the pillow out of the case again and began to run my hands across it to see how many feathers were poking out, and where they were. As I ran my hands across the pillow, my mind began to drift. I know this is crazy but for me, it felt good.

I immediately sat down and found a pair of tweezers and a nail clipper on my dresser. I began to pluck the stems of the feathers that were sticking out of the pillow. What I could not pull out with the tweezers I would cut with the nail clipper. I could feel no more than ten stems, but for me, it gave me a high. It was absolutely crazy, but it was therapy that had excited me.

I felt like I had found an escape in my mind to deal with all that was happening around me. There I was, back in this ball, on the outside, looking in. The feathers were different shades of grey and were different sizes, but most of them were small. There were so many of them, so I knew I could do this for a while. I would then take the feathers and fold them up in a tissue and put them in the trash.

I heard the door open, and I knew that my family had come back. I then took the pillow and hurried to put the case back on it and went downstairs.

James asked me, "How was your time alone?"

I told him it was good and I felt better. Each evening, riding home from work, all my mind could think about was getting home to that pillow. I would come home and take care of what needed to be done for my family then I would say, "James, I am going upstairs to rest."

Before I would go upstairs I would go the pantry and grab a handful of small baggies to take upstairs with me so I could have somewhere to store the feathers as I pulled them out. I would lock the bedroom door behind me so no one could enter. I would then position myself on the bed, find the spot I had marked on the wall, position my eyes on that particular spot, pull the tweezers out, and take the pillow out of the case. I began to run my hands across the pillow to find the feathers that were sticking out. I picked up my tweezers as I began to rock back and forth and hum a tune. It was no special tune, but it was so soothing to me. I was in a world that no one knew but me where I did not have to worry about anyone bothering me, and I could stay there as long as I wanted.

One morning when James got up, he said, "Do you still want me to buy you some new pillows?" I hesitated because I did not want to lose my best friend at the time, which was that pillow, but I told him, "Yes."

He said, "We will throw that one away and get you a better one."

The whole time he was talking I was thinking to myself, *I can hide this somewhere where he will not find it, and I can still have my time with my friend.* I felt if James ever knew what I was doing, he would surely think I had lost my mind.

James brought the new pillows, and I began to sleep on them, but I would lie there, thinking about the other pillow. Late at night when I could not sleep, I would wait until I thought James was in a deep sleep and then would turn my lamp on at my side of the bed and pull the pillow out. I had hidden it inside of my nightstand cabinet where I knew he would not look. I pulled the pillow out and just rubbed my hand across it like always to find the feathers that were sticking up. By now, the pillow had become flatter; I told myself I would have to slow down on pulling the feathers out.

I continued to pluck the feathers almost three nights a week. This went on for a while until one night, I was plucking the feathers and they started to change colors. They appeared to be getting darker; they were no longer grey; instead they were a dark brown, and some of them were jet black. This became scary for me, but I continued to do this. One night, as I started plucking the feathers, James woke up and said, "What are you doing over there?"

I told James that I was clipping my fingernails and my toenails. I had to think of something fast to tell him because I knew he could hear the sound of the nail clipper more then he would hear the tweezers. It was so hard to come to grips with the fact that I knew I was losing my mind. I felt as though I could snap at any moment, but I did not have the courage to tell my husband and family. I could not believe that I was sitting up at night plucking feathers from a pillow that seemed to bring me so much comfort. Something was truly wrong, but my mind did not know how to fix it. The wall that I had built around me to hold me was beginning to crumble. I could no longer keep a steady grip.

One night James woke up and said, "I wake up in the middle of the night and I've seen what you are doing, but I have never said anything. Lillian, what is going on? I know that you are not cutting your nails every night because I see what you are doing to the pillow."

I said, "I'm fine. Please, just go back to sleep."

I immediately put the pillow away and attempted to get some rest. I felt like I had lost the one thing that gave me peace and comfort because James had found out. I felt so bad about lying to my husband again.

The strangest thing was, he let me continue to do it. This one particular night as I met with my best friend, the pillow, I began to pull the feathers out, and this one feather was so hard to pull, but I kept trying to squeeze it through the little opening in the pillow. To my surprise, this ugly "black feather" came out, and it was huge in size, more than the others. The feather frightened me. My mind started to think evil thoughts as though this was a sign of my death.

I told James the next morning, "I don't want to keep doing this; you can throw the pillow away." It was hard for me to come to that decision, but I began to get scared after seeing that big black feather come out of that pillow. It made me realize I had begun to tip over the edge. James wanted to call my family to tell them what had happened, but I said to him, "Please don't tell anyone about this. I just felt like I was in my comfort space when this was happening. This was my way to cope, and I promise it will not happen again."

He embraced me with his strong warm arms and said, "I love you very much, and always know that I am here with you, and I am never going to leave you."

After my intimate relationship with my pillow and plucking its feathers, James said, "I see how this is really affecting your mind."

He finally convinced me to let him tell my family everything that was going on with me. I told him I did not want to put any more worry on my mother because of my father's illness. But in my mind, my heart ached for my mother to be there with me by my side.

James said, "Lillian, it is important that someone else in the family knows what's going on with your health."

I just nodded with my head hung down as I cried.

He told me, "Lillian, I know we have shared the lupus to some degree but now things have taken a turn where we need to tell your family just how bad things are getting, especially now that you are in this bad state of depression."

With my head still hung down, James said, "Lillian, please look at me. I don't want you to hurt yourself or anyone else."

I wiped my eyes as I looked up at him in a small quivering voice and said, "James, I know I know that we need to do something. This is too much for me to handle by myself; I'm trying to be strong for you, me, and our children. I talk to God and I pray every day, but I need to let someone know what's really going on here. You can tell my sister Sandra, but you cannot tell my mother."

He agreed and said he would only tell Sandra. I begged him not to go into any detail about the pillow.

I said, "If she knew I was doing that, I know she would want me to get some counseling right away. She is the only one that I know who will help bring me out of this."

I felt that way because she was, to me, my "personal pastor" and I had shared so many things with her, and I knew she would understand. I sat on the side of the bed as he called my sister on the phone and asked her if she could come to the house one evening. He wanted to talk with her about us. I could not hear what she was saying to him as I sat wondering how much I wanted to tell her.

Once he made the call, he told me what day she was coming, and he said, "Lillian, I want you to be honest and tell her everything that you are feeling so she can help you and pray for you."

I looked him straight in his eyes and I said I would, but there were just some things I could not share.

James looked at me with disappointment in his eyes as he said, "I am trying to help you. I watch you every day going through your own hell, and there is nothing that I can say or do to help you. Do you know how much that hurts me and tears me up on the inside?"

I looked at him with tears in my eyes and said, "I am sorry James but I am in a place that is not pleasant at all for me. James, where I am is so lonely; I feel like I am lost in the wilderness or in the belly of a beast; my life is being eaten away minute by minute. James, you cannot help me. Please, just pray for me that I do not completely lose my mind. Where I am, I don't want anyone else to be. Every day I struggle to keep my sanity. Just pray for me. That is all that I ask. That is how you can help me."

When my sister Sandra came that evening to talk with James and me, we made sure that the children were in bed and asleep.

As she sat down, she began to ask me, "Peewee, how are you feeling?"

I looked slightly away from her and said, "I am feeling fine; I am just a little tired."

James began to talk with her, and he said, "Sandra, she is not fine, and I am concerned about her. The forty milligrams of prednisone that she is taking along with the other medications and the flare-ups that she continues to have are really getting the best of her."

He looked at me and said, "Lillian, I am sorry, but I have to tell her how you are feeling since you are not."

My sister then said, "I know you all have talked with the doctor; is he saying anything new about her condition?"

James said, "The doctor said the increase of the prednisone seems to be maintaining her kidney function for now, but he doesn't know for how long. In the meantime, she is still doing her blood-work every month, and they are watching her creatine closely, so I am praying there will be a change in her condition."

I finally spoke up and said, "I have an appointment in March, and I will ask him if he is going to take me off of the medicines or lower the doses."

James said to my sister, "She has been on this high dosage for six months now, and I have seen her when she was on ninety-five milligrams a day and she could not function. I cannot say I enjoy seeing her suffer like she is. It is hard watching her cry all the time and hearing her saying she feels like she is losing her mind."

I continued to sit there while they talked about the medicines, and then my sister asked me how I felt my mental state was. I blurted out in a loud voice, "I am tired, and I don't care what happens; I am just tired; my mind cannot continue to handle this. Sandra, I feel like I am losing my mind. I don't want you to tell Mama any of this, because I know that she has a lot of things that she is dealing with."

My sister gave me her word that she would not. She got up from the chair and said, "We are going to pray, and we are going to pray believing Almighty God will bring you through and that He will keep you in your right state of mind."

As we gathered together to hold hands, I began to cry, and it seemed like I could not stop crying. I felt like someone besides my husband could hear me and see my feelings.

After she prayed with us, she gave us both a hug and told us to stay encouraged and told me, "Peewee, please call me whenever you feel like you are going somewhere in your mind that you feel is uncomfortable. You have got to hold on and believe God is with you and that He is going to bring you through."

I looked at her as I began to wipe away my tears and said, "Okay, I will."

My sister said, "I want you to begin reading Psalm 139, and I want you to speak verses thirteen through sixteen to yourself. God knows everything that has happened and will happen. He is present in every situation in our lives. I want you to trust him; you have got to trust him."

After my sister left, James came to me and said, "Do you feel any better at all? I want you to know I'm trying to do all that I can to help you because I love you."

I said to him, "I know, but right now I just want to go lie down. I have a long day at work tomorrow, and I know I am expected to get a lot of work off of my desk."

When I went upstairs, all I could think about was how I wished I had my pillow. That pillow gave me comfort and security. I felt when I was plucking the feathers, it was helping me to take out my frustrations about every inch of pain I felt in my body and everything that I wished I could say to people.

Oh, my God, how I wished that I had my pillow. There was something inside of me that just wanted to start a new one, but I promised James that I would not do that anymore. I looked in my closet and there I saw a small travel pillow that I had purchased a while ago.

I told myself, *This is so small. There may not be many feathers in here.* I grabbed it anyway and locked the door. Just as I began to pull out my tweezers, I could hear James walking up the steps. To me, that was a sign that this was not what I needed to do, and if I did, I would surely lose my mind because I was there, at the edge, and all I needed was something else to send me over the cliff.

I began to think about the promise that I had made to James and how I needed to trust him, but most importantly I needed to learn how to trust the Lord like I did before I became ill. I put the pillow in a bag and stuck it back in the closet.

When James came up the stairs, he knocked on the door and told me, "Lillian, unlock the door and let me in."

When I let him in, I said to him, "There is a pillow in the closet in a bag that I need you to throw away in the morning. I went to the closet and I pulled it out, but something besides hearing your footsteps would not let me start on that pillow."

James said, "It was the Lord. He is holding you, and He wants us to trust Him no matter how hard this gets. I want to see you go back to reading your Bible like you did every day before this happened. Remember how you use to read and quote scriptures? You would sing to the Lord, but now I don't see any of that. You would inspire me to trust God when things got rough in our lives."

I said to him, "My joy is gone, and I want it back, along with my mind, but I don't know how to get either back."

He said, "We are going to start praying together as a family like we used to do."

James kissed me good night, and I tried my best to go to sleep without thinking about the pillow. That was something that I knew I needed to let go of if I wanted to move forward in helping myself to heal in my mind. It was hard to stop my mind from running in all different directions that night, and when I did fall asleep, it felt as though it was time to get right back up and prepare my daily routine with the children and then go to work.

During my days at work, my body felt as though it was getting more tired than usual. My doctor had also written a letter to my job to ask that I be allowed to have special parking privileges because of the systemic lupus and the kidney insufficiency attacking my body.

Once I came home from work, I would do what was needed and expected of me as a mother and wife. Maybe it was not always the way my family wanted it to be, but given my frame of mind, I felt it was my best. I would begin to take each day that was given to me as a time to try my hardest to reflect on the good in what I was going through, but I saw no good in any of it. Every time I would attempt to read a Scripture or hum a song, it all came back to the same feelings. *Why am I doing this? This is something I feel in my life that is irreversible.*

I would often ask myself, "Does God really hear me when I pray, and does He see the tears that I cry every day?"

I would tell the Lord, "You let me cry, you let me scream, and you have watched my heart be broken in two. I want to believe you are there. Lord, please send me a sign that this will not last forever, that my life will not always be like "broken glass" that I am trying to glue and piece back together."

As the days lingered, I no longer had my desire for my pillow—not that I did not think about it, but I wanted to try to move forward, because I missed my life. I kept telling myself that I needed something else to cling to in place of the pillow. In the evenings after work, I would tell James that I needed to take a small nap before I began dinner. I would go to my room, get in the bed, and hide my face under the covers. I would cry to myself quietly so no one would know.

I kept telling myself that if I lay buried under the covers long enough, when I got up, my life would be back to normal. The covers were hot, and I was sweating. Maybe I was at the tipping point, but the sweat was like a cleansing, minute by minute, to change what I was feeling. I would finally get up and wash my face, and return to my family as though everything was wonderful.

When I had time alone to myself while I was at work on my lunch break, I kept trying to remind myself of the scripture that my sister had given me to read. I would open my Bible and begin to read, but then suddenly my mind could not concentrate. This voice that was once in my head made me think of all the things that were going on in my life that were negative. I got up from my desk and went to the bathroom. I made sure no one was in there but me. I found a stall close to the wall and I began to hold my hand over my mouth and cry. I knew eventually I had to return to my desk, so I got myself together, piled makeup back on my face—which I had wiped off from the tears—and returned to my desk. It was important that I put the makeup back on my face because of the discoloration and the lesions that were still there. I could not have people constantly staring at me.

Once I returned to my desk, I tried to produce some work before it was time to leave, but I kept looking at the clock because I could not wait to get out of there. I knew at home I could go to my room and hide under the hot covers until the sweat would wash away some of the hurt.

One Saturday morning, I lay in the bed most of the morning thinking and crying to myself. I told myself I needed to bring myself out of this depression but I knew I could not do it alone. After the sweat kept falling, I began to realize, *This is not what you need, and this is not helping you.* So, I got up and got my Bible and I began to read Psalm 139 over and over. I wanted it engraved in my mind because I knew that was the only way I could go on. I had begun to realize through much tears and prayer that I needed to turn to God and trust him to bring me through. I looked out the window and saw the bright sunshine, and something inside of me wanted to feel that on my skin and in my life again.

> *Even though I walk through the darkest valley,*
> *I will fear no evil, for you are with me;*
> *Your rod and your staff, they comfort me.*
> **(Psalm 23:4)**

Chapter 15

FACING DIALYSIS

Over the months, I began going back to church more steadily; I tried to be more open to my friends and family by engaging in conversation with them. I even began to become more involved in my children's school activities as much as I could. James would always go because I said I did not feel well. One morning was a morning like no other morning. I began to realize God does love me and He is here with me. Once again, I started to live my life with so much appreciation for each breath that I could breathe. I would drink plenty of water; I ate as many vegetables as I could. I did my best to stay away from red meat because my doctor said that it was not good for my body with the lupus being so active.

I continued to take my medicines and try to live my life in a way that would help me adapt to the change caused by my illness.

In March of 2001, I left work early to attend my doctor's appointment. As usual, I went in so he could discuss my blood-work. This time, I put myself in a frame of mind not to expect to hear anything different or positive because there was always the same sad news.

The doctor told James and me, "Mrs. Forbes, your kidneys are still maintaining an okay function, but you are still not out of the woods."

After the doctor made that statement, I said, "What else can I do—because I am tired, and I want my life back."

"Mrs. Forbes, you have been through a lot, but you have come a long way. I am going to leave the prednisone dosage where it is, and I will see you back in September."

I looked at the doctor with disappointment and anger at the same time and said, "This prednisone is making me crazy, and I know I have been on a high dosage before, but for some reason, my mind is not adjusting to this."

The doctor said, "Mrs. Forbes, I am sorry, but right now this is where we stand. Let's hope when you return, there is more of a significant change."

We left the doctor's office and came home, and before we picked up our children, James said, "I want you to hang in there because I believe it's going to get better. I believe God has not forgotten us, and I know he hears our prayers."

I looked at him and said, "I believe that, but, how much more will God put on me because I can't take any more."

On September 14, 2001, I had an appointment with my nephrologists and my rheumatologist. I was praying the appointment would go well. This time, I was expecting some good news—better than before—because our wedding anniversary was coming up on the seventeenth. James and I once again walked into the doctor's office in anticipation of nothing but the best. The doctors greeted us both and asked us to please sit down.

The nephrologists immediately asked me, "Mrs. Forbes how are you feeling today?"

I looked at the doctor, thinking he had good news to tell me. I said, "I am feeling fine, just a little tired, and my urine does not seem as clear from the last time I saw you. Is there something wrong?"

The doctor said, "Your creatinine has increased some, so I want you to get your blood drawn every two weeks along with your twenty-four-hour urine test."

I said, "I am drinking plenty of water and still eating all of the vegetables I can."

The doctor said, "Mrs. Forbes, that really does not have much bearing on your kidney function now. The lupus has severely scarred your kidneys, and as I stated before, we are doing everything possible to not go the dialysis route."

By this time, I began to panic, because just hearing the word "dialysis" sent chills up my spine.

The doctor said, "When you do your next labs, we will look at them and talk."

James and I headed home. James said, "Do you still want to go away for the weekend to celebrate our anniversary?"

I said, "No."

He said, "I think we need to go away and just have some time to take all of this in."

Finally, I said okay. We had my family watch our children, and we went away for the weekend to Williamsburg, Virginia, and stayed at a nice quiet bed and breakfast. In my mind, I knew when we returned, this terrible thing that was haunting me would still be in our lives. We had a wonderful time away and did our best not to think about our life in the real world when we returned.

As time moved forward, I tried to move forward with my life. I was still trusting and believing in God that He would change my life for the better. The dark places I found myself in at times were easier to cope with when I would read the Word of God. I found strength and hope in the Scriptures. I reminded myself of some words that I had once written down to myself, which were, "Only God has the blueprints of my life, and only God knows how my life will be."

I continued to pray every day that my kidneys would get better. I would look at Sheree and smile seeing how she was growing up to be so pretty and how she was my miracle baby. I would look at Michelle and tell myself how strong she was, even though I felt like she did not want to be. She showed so much bravery when it came to her mommy being sick. I felt as though she hurt badly for me and she did not understand. It's just a mother's instinct that I could sense about my child.

The months passed, and before I knew it, it was almost Thanksgiving, and then there would be Christmas. It was a time that I would be able to say, "Thank God I am still here." I would be blessed to also see another birthday, so I was anxious to go to my appointment and get some good news.

On October 29, 2001, I had my doctor appointment again to discuss my recent lab results. James and I arrived a little early because we were excited since we had been faithful in our praying and reading the Word. We knew the Lord was going to send us a blessing that day; we felt it. I still drank my water and tried to eat right. I would drink so much water until sometimes I felt like I would float away, even though the doctor had told me that that did not have much bearing on my kidneys.

The doctor had us both to sit down and he began to say, "Mr. and Mrs. Forbes, I would like to reiterate that our main goal here is to do our best to prevent dialysis, and everything we have done so far is working, but it only appears to be helping for a while. What we would like to do is put you back on the drug CellCept."

I looked at him with my mouth open and my eyes focused right into his and asked him, "Why? Doctor I already feel like I am going crazy at times, and it's hard to stay focused."

He began to say, "Mrs. Forbes, I hear what you are saying, but we have to keep trying to see what will work. We are hoping it will bring your creatinine levels down and keep the lupus stable. As I have said before, your creatinine levels have risen, and that is a great concern of mine.

I asked him, "Would the CellCept really help my kidneys this time because I do not want to go on dialysis."

The doctor looked at me with great concern in his eyes and said, "We are going to do our best to make you better. We will continue to do the lab work every three weeks now since you are starting this drug. This way, we will be able to see if there are any changes in your kidneys."

I started taking the CellCept again on November 5, 2001. I did not notice any changes right away to my physical appearance until a month had passed. I noticed my hair began to shed again this time, and there were mild headaches that I would have along with a lot of anxiety. I tried my best to cope with the symptoms because I wanted to make sure I was doing all that I could do to save my kidneys. I continued to go to work every day as though my life was still beautiful. I asked myself, *What can I do but continue to trust God?*

I thought about my birthday and the holidays, wondering how this drug would affect me when I would be around a lot of people. Here I was, still taking the prednisone and feeling zapped out from that every day, and now I would have something new to take.

When my birthday came, I did not want to do anything but stay at home with my family. My energy and self-esteem were so low that I did not want to be around anyone. When the holidays came, my family and I did our best to have a wonderful Thanksgiving and Christmas. When the New Year came in 2002, James and I made a promise to each other that we would do everything we could to keep our family together and put our trust in God. He also asked me if I would try to be more active with my life by getting involved in social activities and get out of the house more besides going to work and church. I told him that I would try but not to expect a lot from me.

I managed to continue to work and try my best to be involved in some social and family activities around me. I spent more time with my family and did fun things with my children on the weekends. Time went by so fast, and I was still doing my lab work for my doctor every three weeks as scheduled. The summer months had come in, and it was hot, so I began to notice swelling more than usual in my ankles. I also noticed swelling in my arms and face. My urine had begun to turn dark; I thought that was unusual because the doctor said I was still maintaining function of my kidneys. I thought the new drug was working. I contacted my doctor because I became worried—I was no longer just concerned. He had me do lab work again because he was concerned now that this swelling appeared to have come so fast over a short period of time.

On May 8, 2002, I went to have my bloodwork done. The doctor said they would contact me as soon as the results were in.

In the evenings, when I would go home, I would lie down and try to get off of my feet. It was hard to rest because the only thing that kept running through my mind was the "D" word: dialysis. I would imagine in my mind all of the shows and movies I would see where people were on dialysis, and it terrified me.

On May 10, which was a Friday, while at work, I remember that morning my supervisor announcing that we would have a fire drill that afternoon, so she wanted us to prepare ourselves to go outside when the time came. I knew it was going to be hot that day, but I wore an olive-green pantsuit with a black shell top and black shoes to work that day. I tried to never wear anything short sleeved in the summer time because I was ashamed of my arms and legs because they were scarred with lesions from the lupus. I went to the cafeteria to eat my lunch, and when I came back, the fire alarm went off. I grabbed my purse and followed everyone else out of the building. I felt so self-conscious because people outside were saying how hot it, was and they were taking off their jackets.

One co-worker said, "Lillian, aren't you hot with that jacket on?"

All I could do was tell her no, but I was actually burning up. When it was time to go back into the building I came in and sat at my desk and noticed my phone was blinking because someone had left me a message. Fear immediately began to sink in.

I took a deep breath and said to myself, *What if this is my doctor? How am I going to react if he gives me bad news over the phone?* I told myself I would go to the bathroom and check my urine to see if it had gotten any lighter, so I did. When I came out of the bathroom, my heart was racing because it had not gotten any better. I went back to my desk and was scared to check the message on the phone.

The phone rang, and it was James, wanting to know if my doctor had called yet with my results. I told him, "There is a message on the phone, and I think it might be him, but I am afraid to call."

He said, "Lillian, check the message and see if it's the doctor. Then, call me back."

When I hung up the phone I took a deep breath, and the tears had already begun to fill my eyes because I knew it was bad news. After what I had been seeing with my urine over the last couple of days, I knew it was nothing positive. I picked up the phone and played the message. It was from my doctor. The words that he said pierced my heart so, until I became cold and still. His message was so stern and direct; I could not take it all in.

"Mrs. Forbes, we have received your bloodwork, and we will need you to come to the hospital to be admitted as soon as you can."

God is our refuge and strength, an ever-present help in trouble.
(Psalm 46:1)

Chapter 16

ACCEPTING DIALYSIS

I sat with the phone in my hand, and all I could hear was a "Beep, beep," before the operator came on. All of a sudden, I burst into tears and my coworkers came rushing to my desk to ask me what was wrong. It took me a while before I could get out what had happened. They immediately contacted James, and he came down to my office.

After they got me to calm down, they asked me, what did the doctor say?

James and I talked with my supervisor to let her know I would probably be taking time off of work for a few weeks or longer. We left for the day and headed home. I cried all the way home and kept saying to James, "What am I going to tell my babies? It is Mother's Day weekend, and I'm supposed to be here with them."

James said, "I know, but right now I have to think about what the doctor is going to tell me when I call him back."

When we got home, we called the doctor back. I apologized to the doctor for taking so long to return his call. James got on the phone and began to ask the doctor what happened. The doctor said, "Her kidneys are just so scarred by the lupus that the medicines

120

were only working to maintain them up to a certain point. Her kidneys are straining to work."

James asked, "Does she have to come into the hospital today?"

"We are waiting on a bed, and as soon as one becomes available, you can bring her in."

I asked, "Could I please come in early Saturday morning because I want to talk to my children. It is Mother's Day weekend, and I know they are going to be sad."

"Mrs. Forbes, you cannot wait past Saturday. Saturday morning, you have to be here in this hospital. When we call you to tell you a bed is ready, you must get yourself prepared to come."

After we hung up, I started screaming to the top of my lungs, telling James that I was scared and did not want to go on dialysis. I began to get sick to my stomach and found myself lying on the bathroom floor. James helped me to get up and washed my face as he tried to comfort me.

He said, "We have got to tell the children, and I know it's going to break their heart, but we have to do it today."

Michelle was on her way home from school, and Sheree would be coming soon. I tried to stop crying, but each time I dried my eyes, I thought about what was happening and would start crying all over again.

I went outside before Michelle came home and stood on my front porch, looking up at the sky. I said, "God, why? Why is this happening to me? Where is my rainbow that you promised me in your Word? God, I want to continue to trust you, but I don't know if I can handle this dialysis. God, I am so afraid—afraid of living with dialysis and afraid of dying. Please God, have mercy upon my soul."

I thought I was getting better. I thought my storm and my time in the wilderness was over. I felt like Job all over again. I felt like I was given a promise that was taken from me. I kept asking myself what I did wrong. *Why am I being put through so much hell and torture?* It felt like torture because each time I would come through one thing, something else would happen, but this felt like the worst blow for me. This time I was surely in the belly of the beast with no way out.

I dried my eyes and went back into the house to wait for my children to come home. The entire time I sobbed and shook my head as I kept repeating over and over to myself, *God, why?* As I sat on the couch in my living room, I heard the door open, Michelle came in.

"Hi Mommy, how do you feel?"

I looked at her with a stare, but no words could come out. As she looked at me, she began to get teary eyed and said, "What's wrong?"

James said, "Michelle, we need to talk to you and Sheree, but we want to talk to you before Sheree comes."

We sat her down and told her, "Mommy has to go back into the hospital, and we don't know for how long."

Then I said to her, "I know it is Mother's Day weekend, but I have to go so the doctors can fix what's going on."

I did not want to tell her about the dialysis. I felt it would be too much for her to handle.

Michelle said, "How are you going to tell Sheree? You know she is going to be upset and start crying."

I said, "I know, so I need you to be strong to help your sister."

Michelle looked at me with big sad eyes and said okay. Sheree was only eight, and I knew it would be hard for her because she was the baby. Even though there was an eight-year difference in age between them, she was doing her best to be brave. She said, "I will make sure that Sheree will be okay."

James got up from the couch and said, "I am going to pick Sheree up from the babysitter, and when I come back, we can tell her. Michelle why don't you come and ride along with me so Mommy can have some time to pack her suitcase?"

She gave me a hug, and they left. As soon as they left, I screamed again and cried. I made myself sick to my stomach because this had taken so much out of me. I couldn't believe this was happening to me. I went from room to room like a crazy person, crying and talking to myself, trying to figure a way out of this maze, but there was none. I had to face the reality that I was going back into the hospital and that I would be going on dialysis. When James and Michelle came back with Sheree, they came upstairs.

I asked Sheree, "How was your day?"

Sheree came to me with that pretty smile and hugged me and said, "Mommy, what you doing? Why are you putting clothes in a suitcase? Are we going away?"

I didn't have the heart to tell her I was going back to the hospital.

James said, "Sheree, slow down. Mommy and I need to talk with you and Michelle."

Just like any eight-year-old, the first thing she said was, "Talk about what?"

I said, "Sheree, come sit on the bed because I need to tell you something, and I want you to listen carefully. Mommy has to go to the hospital tomorrow, and I may be there for a few days."

Then, before Sheree could say anything else, James spoke up and said, "The doctors have to fix Mommy's kidneys, and then she will be back home."

Sheree said, "Daddy, what is a kidney?"

We knew she would not understand, but all we could say to her was the doctors would make me better.

Michelle said, "Sheree, I am going to help Daddy take care of you, and you'd better listen to me." Sheree said, "Okay, Mommy. We will come to see you and bring you back home."

My heart broke for my children. That night, I tried to sleep, but it was hard to do because I did not know what to expect or what would happen to me. In my mind, I kept thinking, *I am not coming back home.*

Finally, Saturday morning came, and the phone rang around ten. It was Georgetown hospital. They said they had a bed and that they would be waiting for me when I arrived. I gave my children a big hug and lots of kisses and told them I loved them.

I said, "I know tomorrow is Mother's Day, but Daddy will bring you up to see me, and I will be home before you know it."

I did my best to be strong for my children because I did not want them to see me fall apart.

When we got to the hospital, they admitted me and assigned me to a room. I lay in the hospital as though I was in another place in time. It all felt make-believe. I watched the nurses come and go and people walk past, but nothing felt like it was my reality. All I could think about was how I looked forward to Mother's Day to spend with my children, but here I was, stuck in this hospital.

The doctor came in and said, "I would like to talk with you both to let you know what we will be doing. We will be watching her urine output for the next few days and will be checking her vitals. She will have to have a shunt surgically implanted to allow for the hemodialysis. We need to do this in order to purify her blood and to remove waste and extra fluid from her body.

"The shunt will be in her upper chest area just above her neck, and the dialysis shunt will hang over her left breast. Mrs. Forbes, you have to be careful how you move around after the shunt is inserted. We will do this surgery on the May 14, and we are going to allow the one day on the fifteenth for your body to rest from the surgery and then we need to start your first dialysis treatment on Thursday the sixteenth.

"Once we do the first treatment, we will see how you and the kidney respond. After we see the labs and look at the bloodwork, and if everything continues to go in a positive direction, you will be getting your treatments three times a week. Her next dialysis treatment will be on Saturday the eighteenth, then the following Tuesday. They will go in that order."

I looked away as he was talking. The doctor tapped me on the foot and said, "Kiddo, I am so sorry; we did everything we could not to get to this point. I am so sorry that things have spiraled downhill, I really am."

I never looked back around at him because I couldn't. I didn't care what anyone said; I was simply there.

James said, "I'm going to go home so I can bring the girls back up to see you since its Mother's Day, and I will call your mom and let her know what's going on. Lillian, please look at me and listen to me: if I could change this for you, I would, and make it all go away, but I can't, and I am so sorry."

He gently kissed me on the forehead and said he would be back.

I never moved from the position I was in. I felt like my life had lost its luster; any means of happiness and joy were all gone. I rehearsed the Scripture of Jeremiah 29:11 in my mind over and over: "For I know the plans I have for you. They are plans for good and not for disaster, to give you a future and a hope."

To me, there was neither for me except for a life of despair. I looked up, and there was a knock on my door; it was the nurse with my lunch tray.

She said, "Mrs. Forbes, how are you feeling? I hope you have an appetite because we need you to eat so your body can be ready for the surgery on the fourteenth." As she put the tray down, she said laid her hand on my arm and said, "Try to eat, and I will be back in a little while."

I looked over at the tray and knew I was hungry, but still I did not want to be bothered with anything. I eventually ate some of my mashed potatoes and a few pieces of sliced turkey in gravy.

A few hours after I ate, James called me on the phone to tell me that they were on their way back. "Sheree is afraid, but I told her it would be okay."

I knew I had to get myself together long enough to put up a front for the children. The nurse came back, got my tray, and said, "I'm glad you tried to eat something. Mrs. Forbes, I see the hurt in your eyes, and I sense you are afraid, but we will do everything we can to make you comfortable and help you with this. Dialysis can be scary for someone who has never experienced it before, but we are here for you."

In my mind, I know she was doing her best to comfort me, but this was my body, and she had no idea how I felt. As I lay facing the wall, waiting on my family to come, I thought about all the different ways that I wished my life could have been different. No matter how hard I tried, I could not understand why this was happening to me. Yet, there was no changing the reality that I was about to face.

Suddenly there was a knock was at the door. I hurried and wiped the tears from my face and tried to put on a big smile as I turned around. James walked over to the bed, kissed me on the forehead, and said, "Happy Mother's Day. How you are feeling?"

Before I could answer, Michelle walked over to me, holding Sheeree's hand. They each had a smile but also had tears in their eyes. They both said, "Happy Mother's Day, Mommy" and they gave me a hug and a kiss. They gave me a gift—a beautiful big crystal clock. My eyes lit up because they said, "We picked it out ourselves."

I asked them, "What made you buy Mommy such a beautiful clock?"

Michelle said, "Because we want you to be our mommy for a long, long time."

Sheree began to cry out loud and started backing away from my bed and said, "My stomach hurts, and I want to go home. I want to go home!"

James and Michelle tried to console her, but I felt she was scared, terrified to see me lying in the hospital bed.

James said, "Let Michelle take you to the bathroom, and then we will leave."

She sniffled and said okay. As they walked out of the room, I said to James, "My baby is afraid of seeing me, and it hurts."

James said. "She just doesn't understand, that's all. I will talk with her when we get home. When they come back, we will leave, and I will call you later, but please don't let this bother you too much."

I told him, "I am trying to take everything in, but knowing that my baby girl is crying because of how she sees her mother on Mother's Day is upsetting to me."

When they came back into the room, James asked Sheree how she was feeling and she said okay, but she wanted to go home.

Michelle said, "She threw up in the bathroom and I asked her if her tummy still hurts, but all she said is she wanted to go home."

James told the girls to give their mommy a hug and kiss and that they would call me later. Michelle came to the bed and hugged me and said, "Mommy, I love you," but Sheree just waved. After they left, I cried myself to sleep.

The next morning, the doctor came in to see how I was feeling and said, "I want you to try to drink a lot today and eat your food because tomorrow your surgery is scheduled for eight o'clock, and you will not be able to have anything to eat or drink after midnight tonight."

After the doctor left, the nurse came in to draw my blood and said they'd bring breakfast shortly. I called James on the phone to let him know what the doctor said so he could be here for my surgery. At this point, I was just going along with everything that I was being told because all the fight I thought I had in me was slowly, slowly leaving.

James arrived at the hospital the next morning around seven. He said, "I wanted to be here early so I could reassure you that you are going to be okay, and I want to pray with you too. Your mom and your sisters and brothers send their prayers and love."

I looked at him with a half-smile and said, "Okay."

Shortly after the nurses came in to get me to wheel me to surgery. While I was riding down the hall, I looked around at everything as if it were my last look. They rolled me into the operating room, and my heart began to pound as if I had a drum inside of me.

The doctor smiled and said, "Good morning, Mrs. Forbes, and how are you feeling?"

I did not answer.

He began to say, "We are going to give you some medicine by IV that will make you sleepy, but when you wake up everything will be done. Remember, you will have a tube inserted in your neck area and two small tubes will be hanging over your left breast, and these tubes will be your port so you can receive your dialysis."

I looked at the doctor through my tears and said, "I'm scared," and started to cry. The doctor kept reassuring me that I would be fine. Not only did they give me medicine to make me sleepy, but they gave me an anxiety pill to calm me.

When I came back to my room, I was a little groggy from the anesthesia, and I began to feel my neck. James said, "Lillian, please don't touch that. You'll have to be careful how you move around."

I felt my breasts, and I could feel two small tubes hanging down from them and I said, "James, what is this?"

He said, "This is the tube that the doctor was telling you about." Then he got a hand mirror and let me see what everything looked like on my body. I just wept because I felt like my body had been violated—it looked so ugly. He said, "The doctor said the swelling will go down soon along with the soreness and some of the bruising."

I lay speechless, looking at the wall in front of me, wanting to disappear right through it.

I know what it is to be in need, and I know what it is to have plenty. I have learned the secret of being content in any and every situation, whether well fed or hungry, whether living in plenty or in want. I can do all this through him who gives me strength.
(Philippians 4:12-13)

Chapter 17

LIVING ON THE BIG MACHINE

The nurse came in a few hours later and said, "Mrs. Forbes the surgery went well, and you will feel better soon. We do have your labs back, and we will be starting your first hemodialysis the day after tomorrow in the morning."

I looked at her and barely got out the words to say, "But I just came from having this thing put in me, and you want to take me back again for something else?"

She said, "Your bloodwork came back late yesterday, and we checked it again this morning along with your urine output. We have to start dialysis soon, but we want your body to have a day of rest first. I am so sorry."

Then she walked out with her head hung down.

I said to James, "I don't want to do this. Why can't I just stay on the medicines?"

James said, "Baby, the medicines are not working. Your kidneys are failing, and I don't want to lose you. You have to take the dialysis. I have to go out for a minute to find the doctor and will be back."

I could tell he was upset and that things had gotten the best of him. Later, he came back and said, "I talked to the doctor, who reassured me everything was going to be fine. He did say since it would be your first treatment, it would take your body time to adjust, but I will be here with you. I'm going to leave now so you can get some rest; know that I love you and will be here in the afternoon."

James left, and I tried to rest, but I could not. All I could think about was how the day after tomorrow would be, what it would it feel like, and if I would come through this. I looked up at the ceiling and I said, "God, please help me. You know I am scared, and you know all of this is hurting me, and my heart is broken." That was all my mouth could speak because I was physically, spiritually, and mentally exhausted.

The next day, I tried my best to rest as they told me to do; James came to see me on his lunch hour and stayed to eat with me. He said, "When I leave work, I will make sure you can talk to the children before they go to bed—especially Sheree."

I said. "Okay, because I want to hold her and comfort her, but I can't; she won't let me."

James said, "Don't worry; that will change over time once you are home and she sees you are fine."

He kissed me and said, "I will be here early for your first treatment, and if they let me hold your hand, I will," and then he left.

Later that evening, the doctor and the nurse came back in to talk with me about the dialysis treatments. They went over in detail again everything they would be doing, and how I would feel after dialysis, and what I should expect. I listened, but it went in one ear and out the other. After they left, I ate most of my dinner—as much as I could—and felt like it would be my last meal ever. I tried to sleep that night, but I couldn't. I wanted to lash out at someone, but there was no one to lash out at.

I lay all night on my pillow, which was cold and damp from crying all night, until it was morning. Before I could do anything, the doctors were at my door, and James was behind them. It was as though a group of monsters had come to get me and take me away to a place where I would never see anyone I loved again.

James said, "I am here, and it's going to be okay."

They wheeled me into a big operating room where I saw big strange machines. I began to cry, and the doctor said, "Mrs. Forbes, we need you to remain calm so your blood pressure will not go up." There was a big machine that looked like a refrigerator with a long tube wrapped around the front of it, and as I got closer the front, it looked like a dryer. They explained to me that this was the machine that would be used for dialysis. They checked my vitals before they started, and then I lay there while the nurse uncovered my left breast. I felt like I was being stripped of any type of dignity that I once had. This machine took all of my self-esteem that I had left; it was taking any hopes of me wanting to go on away. I so badly wanted someone to come and save me, to pick me up and carry me away to a safe place, but there was no one.

The nurse began to take a big thick tube connected to the machine and hooked it up to the tube hanging from my breast. I asked her, "What are you doing to me?" in the midst of my tears.

She said, "We will be starting in a few minutes, and you are going to hear a loud noise. Your body may feel awkward, but we are here with you."

I was sniffling and asked if James could hold my hand, and they said only for a few minutes. James walked over to the bed and held my hand until the machine came on. The machine was so loud that I felt like monsters were taking me away, but all I could do was lie there. I began to scream; my body became cold, and I began to vomit. I could hear the doctor saying, "Her blood pressure is dropping too low." I could hear the doctor telling James, "Please step to the side," but I did not want him to let go of my hand and leave me there.

I looked at James while he stood helpless with tears in his eyes, and I began to cry out, "I want my mother here! James, I want my mother."

James looked at me and nodded, saying, "Lillian, your mom cannot be here. Please let the doctors do what they need to do." I felt like my life was being sucked out of me, and the pains in my legs were so bad, all I could do was continue screaming. I looked at the machine, and I saw blood going around the big tube. I just knew they were draining me of any chance to live that I had left.

I stayed on that machine for two and half hours, which felt like torture and pain. After it was over, they wheeled me back to my room where I slept most of the day. When I woke up, I felt like I had been through a complete carwash cycle and a washing machine cycle and sent through the wringer. My body was extremely exhausted. I had pain in my stomach, which brought me to tears. They gave me something mild for the pain so I could try to eat something. James sat by my bed without much to say.

The doctor came in to remind me again that my next treatment would be on Saturday around the same time.

I said to him, "My body feels terrible, so how can I have another treatment so close? I am still trying to gain my strength back."

The doctor said, "Mrs. Forbes, this is how the treatments are administered. We will have a social worker to come in and talk with you on next week before you are discharged."

I asked him, "Why do I need a social worker?"

He said, "Because you are now a patient with renal failure, and because you will be on Medicare, we have to set up your treatments at a facility close to your home. Please don't worry about that today; try to get some rest."

This was all too much for me; I didn't even know what my thoughts were about anymore.

James sat with me for a while, then he had to return to work.

When Friday night came, I dreaded having to wake up on Saturday morning. They came bright and early to get me to take me to dialysis. I wanted James there, but he could not come. I felt alone, as if I was dying with no family around. Someone was supposed to be there to save me. There I was, this frail person, just going through the motions of dying a slow death with no lifeline to save me. I kept asking myself, *God, where are you, where are you?*

I repeated my dialysis at Georgetown that following Tuesday, Thursday, and Saturday. The treatments never got any better. I was always extremely tired and felt sick to my stomach each time. I would lie in bed or try to sit up on the side, always drooling from my mouth. There always seemed to be excessive saliva in my mouth. I asked the nurse about it, and she said that it was one of the side effects some patients experience in the beginning of their treatments.

Later that Saturday afternoon, the social worker came in to visit me and talk with me about my treatments following my being released from the hospital. She wanted to make sure of my complete address so she could check to see which facility was close to my home.

After we talked about the facility she found, she said, "I will call the facility, which is Fresenius Kidney Care in Waldorf, Maryland, to let them know when to expect you and that you will be a new patient under their care. I will need to let them know that you have chronic renal failure due to your lupus."

The only silver lining I saw out of this was my doctor has other patients at the facility so I would be able to see him once a week. I tried to find something to give me some hope because I had none.

I continued my treatments the Thursday of that week and I was given special instructions from the doctor and nurses before I was released. They said I would be reporting to the new facility on May 28 to start my first treatment. The morning that I was released from the hospital was Sunday, May 26. I was scared to go home, and I was scared to see my children now that I had this ugly tube in my neck hanging over my breast. I did not know how my family would react when they saw me. I felt like a stranger going home to my own family.

When James and I got home, my children looked at me with tears in their eyes. Michelle said, "Hi Mommy," and went straight to her room. Sheree never came near me, so James took her upstairs with Michelle. I stood in the middle of the floor crying because my own children were afraid of me and did not kiss or hug me.

James came back downstairs and said, "Lillian, you have got to give them time."

I said, "Just take me upstairs so I can be alone." There was nothing for me to do but lie on the bed, careful of which way I moved because of the shunt in my neck.

James brought my suitcase up to me and said, "I need to call your mom and let her know you are home."

I told him, "Don't bother because I don't want to see anyone, and I don't want to talk to anyone."

He said, "I, at least, have to let her know you are here."

As I lay on the bed, a knock came to my door, someone sniffling and sobbing. I looked over toward the door and saw it was Michelle standing in the doorway holding Sheree's hand. She said, "Mommy are you okay? We didn't mean not to hug you, but we are scared."

I told Michelle, "I understand," as I held back my tears, "Please bring Sheree over to me," but Sheree cried and said, "I don't want to. I'm scared," and ran back into her room.

I told Michelle to go and be with her and that I would be okay. Oh, how that crushed my heart so bad. I felt like I had nothing to live and no reason to put this hurt and pain on my children.

Later that evening, James fixed me something to eat, but I did not have an appetite. I had to be careful of my fluid intake, so I tried not to eat or drink a lot.

My mother called me on the phone, and when I said hello, I burst into tears and said, "Mama, I can't do this. I am tired and am scared, and I don't want to do this anymore."

My mother was trying to be strong for me by holding back her tears, but I could tell by her voice that she was crying; all she kept telling me was I was going to be okay, and that God was with me.

She then said to put James on the phone. I handed James the phone and I heard him tell her that he would call her back.

Monday was my day of rest to prepare my body for the new facility on Tuesday. On Tuesday morning, James stayed home from work to take me. When I arrived, I was greeted by three nurses and technicians. They told James to come back to get me in four hours. My heart immediately began to race and I looked at the nurse and said, "Why are you saying 'four hours'?"

The nurse said, "Mrs. Forbes, when you were in the hospital you were only given dialysis on the machine for two-and-a-half hours a day because you were just starting your treatments, but now this will be an ongoing procedure because your kidneys are just not working, so you will be on the machine for four hours each time you come."

My mind began to feel jumbled with confusion; voices told me if I could not take the pain two-and-a-half hours, then how I could survive for four hours? I looked at the nurse and said, "I can't do this, please, I can't do this."

The nurse said, "Mrs. Forbes we are going to take good care of you."

They wheeled me back into a room that had at least twelve beds on each side of the walls. I looked around and saw I was the youngest person in there. There were gigantic ugly steel machines with big tubes circled in the front of them. I saw blood circulating through the tubes on all the machines. They were different from the ones in the hospital because they were so huge. I wanted to get up out of my chair and run out of there, but I knew I couldn't.

I felt violated all over again by people I did not know.

They put me in a bed and began hooking the tube from the big machine to the tube on my breast. I just lay there and let them do whatever they wanted to me because I felt helpless; there was nothing I could do. The machine started to turn on, and my body began to feel sick again. I felt like the life was being sucked out of me once more. I lay still as I watched my blood being filtered through the machine. I have never been raped, but I felt like I was being raped over and over by this machine as everyone watched. I let out a loud scream because my legs began to get awful muscle cramps.

The nurse came over and began to massage my legs as I lay crying. She said, "Sometimes they take too much fluid off, and that is how you get these muscle spasms."

After she massaged my legs, the pain went away, but they were sore. To me, four hours could not come fast enough. The nurses gave me headphones to use so I could play music or watch television to pass the time. No matter what she did, it was not enough to take this away from me.

When James came to get me, I could hardly walk because I was so exhausted from the treatment. When I got home I became sick to my stomach again and I went straight to bed. When my children came home, they only stuck their heads in my bedroom door. Michelle said hi, but Sheree still never said a word.

Memorial Day weekend was coming up when we always did things as a family, but this time was different: we were home. James and the children were in the backyard putting hotdogs and hamburgers on the grill, and I was in the bed.

My mother, sister, and brothers came to see me that weekend. When they saw me, I could see the hurt in their eyes to see me with the tube in my neck. They tried to hide their feelings, but I could see their hurt for me.

I remain confident of this: I will see the goodness of the
Lord in the land of the living.
Wait for the Lord; be strong and take heart and wait for the Lord.
(Psalm 27:13-14)

Chapter 18

STILL HOLDING ON

I continued the hemodialysis for six months. My mother or my neighbor would take me three times a week for my treatments because James still had to work. After each treatment, I would come home with pure exhaustion not wanting to eat but just wanting to lie down and sleep. My body started to get frail, and my weight was 105 pounds. My skin began to turn dark and ashy in color. I developed sores around my mouth from the lupus and the dialysis. I felt like the ugliest person there was, but I held on to a thread of hope, believing that in all that I was going through, God had not forgotten about me. My skin began to itch badly, and I began to get different black spots on my body, almost similar to the lupus lesions. The doctor told me it was from the dialysis, and he gave me some cream to stop the itching.

My doctor would come into the facility and check on me every week and do bloodwork to see how I was doing and to see how my body was adjusting to the hemodialysis. At one of my treatments, he said he needed to talk with my husband and me when James came to pick me up.

I asked him, "What's wrong?"

And he said, "I will talk with you both when he comes."

I began to worry because I felt like something was going wrong that he was not telling me.

On my next treatment day, I was totally exhausted when James came to pick me up, and all I wanted to do was go home and get in bed.

The doctor came in before I left and said, "Now is a good time to talk to you both."

The doctor sat down and began to tell us, "The hemodialysis is not filtering the toxins out of your blood as much as we would like. Your body is weak, and I think this type of dialysis treatment is too much for you."

James looked at the doctor with a puzzled look as I sat in silence.

The doctor said, "What we would like to do is start your wife on the home dialysis, which is called the peritoneal dialysis. What we would do is an in-and-out surgery and remove the shunt from her neck. Instead, she would have to have a peritoneal catheter placed in her abdomen."

I said, "Why do you have to keep doing all of these things to me?"

The doctor said, "Mrs. Forbes, we want to help you and give you a better quality of life, and I think this is the way to go. I am certain that you want to return to work at some point, and if you are on this type of dialysis you can return to work and be excused at a certain time during the day. This will allow you to do your dialysis exchanges. I really think that this is the way to go for you."

I had the surgery, and they placed the catheter in my abdomen. As I looked down at my breast, which was swollen and scarred from the shunt, I began to look at my stomach, which was so sore, causing me pain. I still could not believe that I would be leaving this facility with a tube in my abdomen. I was numb and empty on the inside. I felt like I was a leaf that had fallen off its tree limb, and whichever way the wind blew, that's where I was going. I was in a daze and had nothing to add to the conversations going on around me. I came home after the surgery and was adjusting to the tube in my abdomen. Later that week, the dialysis facility contacted me to schedule a date for the machine to arrive.

A few days later, the dialysis nurse came to my home and brought the peritoneal dialysis machine that would be providing dialysis for me every night along with a video to show us. She also brought a few bags of dialysis solution for the machine until my supplies came. She informed us that I would have a truckload of supplies that would come every month with my solution. The nurse set up the machine in my bedroom right beside my bed and put the two bags of solution on top of the machine. She explained that the top of the machine served as a warming pad. She also let us know that the warming pad was needed because cold dialysis solution can cause severe cramping. She said, "Tonight you will start your first treatment at home, and I want you to be careful and wash your hands and put on your face mask. Anybody who comes into the room while you are on this machine has to wear a mask and a gown for the first few months, because we do not want to risk a chance of infections."

I nodded, because things were coming at me so fast and it was just too much to take in at one time. That night, I started my first treatment. I was nervous and scared. James put the two bags of solution on the warming tray as I lay in bed, waiting to be connected to this machine. One thing that I had to understand was that there would be a schedule for me to follow.

James explained to the girls what would have to take a place and once again, he said, "Mommy is going to be fine."

I had to trust God like never before, because this was the worst blow for me to adjust to. As I lay in the bed next to my loving husband with this long tube hanging out of my stomach attached to this machine every night, I felt less and less like a wife or a woman. Although James kept telling me he loved me, I knew in my heart it had to be hard for him to see me like this, because it was hard for me to even look at myself. My husband stayed by my side while I was on the dialysis machine. Every night he would make sure that the machine was working properly and that I was okay. I would look at him and think, *This is what makes me love him even more*.

I knew the day would come when I would return to work and take my dialysis solution and supplies with me. I dreaded that day. The first day the truck came to bring my supplies, I was in total shock to see so many boxes at one time. There were sixty boxes of dialysis fluid, an IV pole, disposable bed pads, sterile masks, scissors, gauze tape, and a scale. I had to store all sixty boxes in my empty bedroom, and there were so many that they were stacked up to the ceiling.

When I returned to work, I had to explain to my supervisor my health situation and how it had become more crucial and severe. I had a blue duffle bag on wheels, which I packed my supplies in each morning before I left for work. There were so many mornings that I would go to work late because the dialysis would make me sick at night. I had so many episodes of fluid buildup around my heart and vomiting throughout the night. My husband would have to rush me to the emergency room until they got things under control. My life was on hold because there was nothing that I could do. I felt like a prisoner in my own home. My husband and I could no longer do anything together as a married couple. I would often think about when we were so happy and able to have date nights together, but now we were just holding on to a hope that was thin.

The dialysis was draining me, and I would constantly have to be on the machine for four hours then off the machine for two hours.

Once I got back on the machine for the evening, I would have to stay on it all night until the morning. In the morning, I would cry and say to James, "I do not feel like going to work today."

James would say, "I know, but you have to go. While we are waiting for the truck to come with your supplies, try to lie back down for a few minutes and eat some crackers so you can feel better."

After the truck came, I would gather my belongings and go to work, and once I came home, I had a few minutes to spend with my children until it was time to go on the machine.

My nurse came out once a month to check on the machine and me; she also would examine the site area where the catheter was inserted. She said, "Mrs. Forbes, you are doing a great job in keeping the area clean; I do not see any infection, so that is a good thing."

This would go on for months—the same routine over and over every day, the routine of the doctors, the medicines, and the dialysis. I didn't care about life anymore. This dialysis machine dictated my world and my life. I missed out on so many family gatherings and things in life that were special to me. Each time my children wanted to go somewhere or do something, I could not go because I did not feel well. James was such a wonderful husband and father because he would do everything he could to shelter them and let them know their mommy would be better soon.

So many days I spent my life in my bedroom looking at the walls and that machine. During these times, my mind would drift back to my old best friend, my pillow, and pulling those feathers out one by one. I kept telling myself as I lay there, day in and day out, that there is a blessing in this somewhere from God. I was reading one day and this paragraph caught my attention. It said, "If you saw the size of the blessing that was coming your way, you would understand the magnitude of the battle you are fighting."

The Lord is my strength and my shield; my heart trusts in him, and
he helps me.
My heart leaps for joy, and with my song I praise him.
(Psalm 28:7)

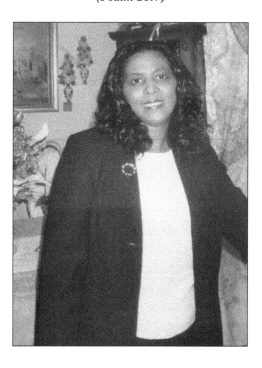

Chapter 19

THE SECRET PLACE OF GOD

One Sunday as I sat in my church crying, my nephew wrote me a letter on the back of his church bulletin. This letter was so powerful because it expressed so much love and faith. It convinced me that I knew that I had to start trusting God with everything that I had. His letter touched my heart so, and these are the words that gave me the encouragement and hope to continue to fight and press my way. His letter said,

> *Hold on. Help is on the way . . . as a matter of fact, it is already here.*
>
> *I know that you know this but, still I say to you that this battle/war/fight is not yours to worry about. I know that you love the Lord and you trust in Him, but I still want to say to you that Jesus is still in control. Peewee, I love you truly and I care for you, and I know that I have never been through what you've been through. But I know it in my heart that God will deliver you. But!! You can't do no more than to trust and obey. Your faith will surely see you*

*through. Remember Job. God will see you through,
I promise you.*

*Love ya always.
Boo ☺ July 1995*

I began to look at my situation differently over time, and I began to thank God for each day he gave me, no matter how hard it was for me. I did my best to make every day count in a good way.

On June 23, 2004, I had an appointment to see my doctor for a follow-up for the lupus and to see how the peritoneal dialysis was working for me. The doctor was pleased with my numbers and was glad that I could have a better quality of life. He also asked, "How are you feeling in all of this?"

I said to him, "I am having some stiffness and pain in my lower legs and feet. Each morning, when I get up, it is hard to stand on my feet, and my knees ache badly."

The doctor said, "I see you have more lesions that have appeared on your skin. We will watch them to see if we will need to do a biopsy on one of them. I feel the stiffness is coming from the inflammatory and degenerative arthritis related to your lupus. We will recommend that you see an orthopedist if the pain gets any worse. In the meantime, I will give you a prescription for the pain and see how this helps. Mrs. Forbes, I would like to see if we can work toward putting you on the list for a kidney transplant. I am suggesting this because your body is adjusting to the peritoneal dialysis, and the lupus appears to be somewhat calm at this time."

I looked at him in such amazement and said, "That never crossed my mind."

My heart began to flutter with excitement, and all I could think about was having my normal life back. I had been on dialysis since May 16, 2002, which was two years and two months, and now it was June 2004. Just the idea of maybe having a life again and being a wife and a mother was more joy to me than anyone could ever imagine.

The doctor said, "You would have to be placed on a waiting list at three different hospitals just in case a kidney becomes available.

In order to get started, there are several tests we would have to perform on you to make sure your body is strong enough for the operation. Once everything comes back and the test looks good, we will add your name to the list. Also, when you are on the list, a lot of times you will receive a cadaver kidney."

I looked at him and said, "What is that?"

He said, "That is a kidney of someone who is deceased, but the kidney may be in good condition."

I sat there frozen, thinking crazy thoughts of how I did not want someone else's kidney in me if they were deceased. However, I tried to convince myself that I would have a chance of no longer being on dialysis.

"Please keep in mind, Mrs. Forbes, sometimes you are on the waiting list for six months to a year before a match is found. I know you have a large family of nine siblings. I wanted to ask you if you would be willing to talk your family to see who would want to be tested to give you a kidney. If they agree to be tested and if someone is a match, there will be a series of tests that we would have to run on them also."

I looked at my doctor and said, "This never crossed my mind. I was not sure if I would even qualify for a transplant because of the lupus."

He said, "I understand, and sometimes we do not offer this because there are times when major surgery is done that can cause a lupus flare-up. However, you are adjusting to the medicines and the dialysis, so now would be a good time. We would have to do a complete workup on you to make sure the lupus is stable, and you will be put on the lists for Georgetown University, Washington Hospital Center, and Johns Hopkins. If you are receiving a cadaver kidney, we try to choose a hospital that you will have time to come to when the kidney is available. But if one of your family members is a match, we would schedule a date and time to have the surgery done. Once you leave today, try to talk with your family to see who is willing to be tested. Please know that this will be a big decision for them to make and that this is major surgery. I do not want you to be disappointed if for some reason even though they are your family, they may be hesitant to donate. You can call me next week after you talk with your family to see if anyone is willing to be tested. One of your relatives may very well be a match.

"I want to let you know there are important determining factors for a transplant to be successful. The antibodies in the blood have to match almost exactly in order for the kidney to function properly. It would be wonderful if we were able to match you with a family member who was not a smoker, does not have high blood pressure, and did not drink alcohol. By doing this, we would not have to be concerned with giving you a cadaver kidney, which could sometimes cause rejection over time. It's always a more successful chance of the transplanted kidney adjusting better to your body when it comes from a family member."

I said to him, "I will go home and talk with my family, and I will get back to you."

When we got up to leave, I looked at the doctor and said, "Doctor, I never thought this was possible for me, and I thought I would be on dialysis for the rest of my life."

I hugged him before I realized what I was doing. The doctor said, "Mrs. Forbes, I am happy that you are adjusting to everything that is going on in your life. I know it has been hard for you, but continue to hang in there because things are looking so much better."

When I got in the car, all I could say was, "Thank you Jesus for hearing my cry and seeing my tears."

Even though I had not talked to my family yet, a sense of peace came over me, and I began to cry with a grateful heart.

Once we came home, James and I talked with Michelle and Sheree to tell them what the doctor wanted to do. Michelle understood a little, but Sheree was still standoffish when it came to me. As time went on, she began to get better, and we began to build on a strong mother-and-daughter relationship.

We told them we didn't know when this could happen, but I would have to talk to their aunts and uncles to see who would be willing.

Michelle spoke up and said, "Mom, I will give you one of my kidneys."

I looked at her with joy in my eyes and said, "Michelle that is so sweet, but you are too young, and you are just beginning to live."

She said, "Mommy, suppose no one wants to give you a kidney."

I told her, "It is in God's hands now, and he will work it out."

I felt God had already made a way for me. As time went on, I spent more time in the Word of God as He drew me closer to Him. I felt that He was giving me a new opportunity for life, and I had to be willing, obedient, and ready to walk completely with Him without hesitation.

When the weekend came, I called my mother to tell her I wanted to have a family meeting with my siblings to discuss the possibility of someone being a match to give me a kidney. My mom was excited and concerned at the same time. She did not want me to get my hopes up if no one was a match.

We all met on June 26, and I shared everything with them—as much of what the doctor had told me. I told them where they could go to have the test done, and if they were a match and willing, the doctors would contact them. I also had to let them know it takes several months for the results to come back. My brothers and sisters said that they would make arrangements to be tested to see if any of them were a match.

My nephew looked at me when we were talking, but he never openly said he would get tested. He has always been a person with a big heart but isn't vocal about his feelings. He is just one of those special people that God created.

That was a happy day for me to know that one of them could possibly be a match to give me a kidney. I knew that my family loved me very much and that they were tired of seeing me sick and in pain.

As the months went by, I was still going to work and doing my peritoneal dialysis every day; it seemed to become better as the days went on because I could see a silver lining in the clouds for me. Though the waiting game was hard to see who a match would be, I stayed focused on my walk with the Lord. I began to know him as my Savior, the one who died for me. I began to understand that He had never left my side, but all I had to do was to trust Him and have faith. The Bible tells us that God can and will do the impossible, and I believed just that.

As my walk grew stronger along with my faith I began to finally understand this was all in God's plan for my life. I would call the doctor every other month to see if there was any good news about the blood tests.

The nurse at the doctor's office told me, "Mrs. Forbes I know you are anxious, but this type of testing is involved and takes time. I will tell you some good news; a family member just may be a match because they have your exact blood type. I am not sure which family member it is. We are still running several tests to be certain. It will take several months before we get the entire test back."

I tried to stay calm, but there was so much happiness inside of me until it was hard to think about anything else. It was now the beginning of October, and I never had to wait so long to hear news that would change my whole life. Finally, I received a letter on October 6 informing me that I had to come into the hospital on October 11 for a preoperative examination for the surgery. I went in and had the examinations done and other testing that was needed. I still had not received the final word yet as to whether or not any of my family members would be an exact match. While sitting at my desk on October 18, my doctor called and said, "Mrs. Forbes, I have wonderful news for you. We have a match for your transplant."

I thought he meant a match from the list that I was placed on, so I said to the doctor, "Are you saying you have a cadaver kidney that is a match?"

The doctor said, "No, the match is one of your family members. The young man who will be giving you your kidney is your nephew; he is a perfect match. You have the same antibodies and the same blood type."

All I could do was scream with excitement. I started crying and kept saying, "Thank you Jesus." I completely forgot where I was, but it did not matter to me. After I calmed down, I asked my doctor if they had contacted my nephew, and he said they had just finished talking with him and explained to him the series of test he would have to do.

The doctor said, "Your nephew is more than willing to give his kidney. Please go and share this wonderful news with your husband and family, and I will be talking with you soon."

I had such wonderful and caring doctors who took good care of me, and they always made sure I understood everything that they were doing to make me better.

My phone rang again; it was my nephew. I said, "Boo, I can't believe that you are a match to give me a kidney."

I kept thanking him over and over again as I was crying. We both chuckled on the phone and said we would see each other later.

After I got off the phone with my nephew, I immediately called James on the phone. We were both so happy and thankful. James and I could not believe that my nephew was a perfect match. My nephew is Daryl (Boo) Hall, the oldest son to my sister Pastor Sandra Smith, and I owe all of my happiness to God and him. My nephew was an auto mechanic, and it never crossed our minds that it would be him. He is a deeply religious person whose belief in God is strong, and he shared with me that God told him that he would be the one that God would use to heal his aunt.

I called my mom and the rest of my sisters; I wanted to tell the whole world what God had done for me and how he used my nephew to be the blessing. My mind immediately went back to the letter he had written to me in 1995 on the back of a church bulletin encouraging me to hold on.

I believe God was preparing him and preparing me, but I could not see my way. My nephew has rheumatoid arthritis, but yet he still wanted to give me his kidney without a second thought.

To me, that was truly unconditional love.

My family was so happy for me, and my children were so glad to know they would be getting a brand-new mommy. Our surgery was scheduled for October 25, 2004 at Johns Hopkins Hospital. We had to be there that morning at 6:00 A.M. to be prepped for the surgery. There were fourteen family members, including my pastor, who spent the day in the waiting area of the hospital during our surgery.

The doctor came out and said, "My God, I have never seen such a wonderful support system."

My nephew and I lay in the same room on beds across from each other; we had some family members in there with us before we went to surgery. We laughed and told a few jokes, and we all had prayer and said we loved each other.

I have learned God's love cannot be measured or limited by how great or how little we may suffer; His love teaches us that nothing can separate us from His love. We had the surgery on October 25, 2004, and we were released from the hospital after a week.

After the surgery, I had to receive outpatient pulmonary treatments for my lungs at Washington Hospital Center in Washington, DC for an entire year. These treatments were given in order to prevent any type of pneumonia from getting into my lungs. I was on a heavy regiment of pain medication and prednisone. But thanks be to God, we made it.

At the time of this writing, it's been twenty-three years since my lupus diagnosis, and I still go to Johns Hopkins every two months to have my blood checked and to be seen by my doctors. My medicines have decreased to five pills a day, which includes two types of anti-rejection medicines, which I will be taking for the rest of my life.

My nephew is doing fine, and we are closer than ever. God has me on a journey, and He is still walking with me on this path called life. God is head of my life, and He is in charge of my life. I am a living witness for others to see our God is a healer and a deliverer. I stand on the Scripture today found in Job 23:10: "But he knows the way that I take; when he has tested me, I will come forth as Gold."

I have learned through this journey that God's love is irreplaceable because it is a true love. I know I have to keep pressing my way, realizing I can't look behind me anymore to wonder what could have been, or what I thought I could change. I needed the Lord, and I needed to be still before him. His power and his presence are awesome, and when the Lord speaks to us, we are to listen and obey. I have learned from reading the Word of God that there are two paths of life that are before us: God's way of obedience or the way of disobedience. This day and forever I choose to follow and obey the Lord, for he has been so merciful and gracious to me.

I thank God every day for my nephew and his obedience and his unselfish love.

But he knows the way that I take; when he has tested me, I will come forth as gold.
My feet have closely followed his steps; I have kept to his way without turning aside.
I have not departed from the commands of his lips; I have treasured the words of his mouth more than my daily bread.
(Job 23:10-11)

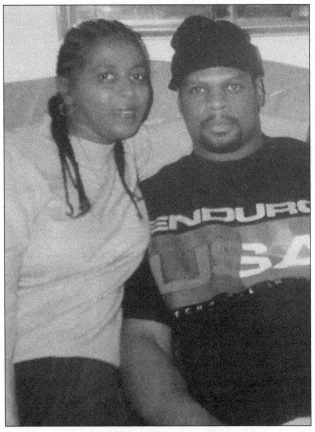

Mrs. Lillian M. Forbes (left)
Mr. Daryl "Boo" Hall, nephew (right)

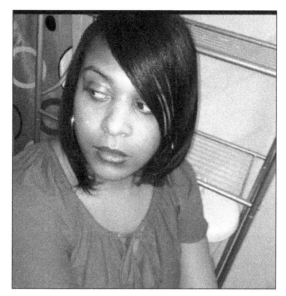

Michelle R. Forbes

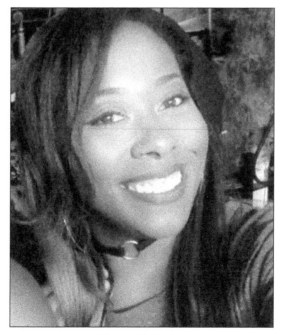

Sheree N. Forbes

EPILOGUE

I n Isaiah 38:4–7, King Hezekiah became ill to the point of death. Hezekiah turned his face to the wall and prayed to the Lord as he wept bitterly. The Lord said to him, "I have heard your prayer and seen your tears; I will add fifteen years to your life. This is the Lord's sign to you that the Lord will do what he has promised."

What the Lord did for King Hezekiah, he has done for me. I pray my story will encourage someone to know almighty God is true to his word.

Today I continue to walk in the footsteps that God has placed before me through the ministry he has given me. God says in His word in Isaiah 43:1–2:

> But now this is what the Lord says he who created you, "Do not fear, for I have redeemed you; I have called you by name, you are mine. When you pass through the waters I will be with you; and when you pass through the rivers they will not sweep over you. When you walk through the fire you will not be burned. The flames will not set you ablaze."

I knew if I had gone in my own strength, I would have drowned, for God showed me grace and mercy.

Through this triumphant journey, God has healed me in mind, body, and spirit. To Him I give honor, glory, and praise!

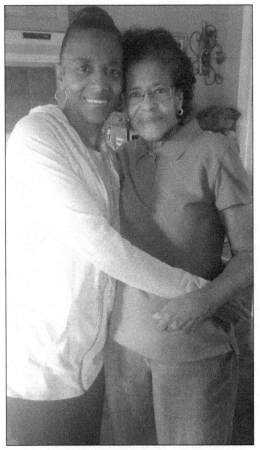

Mrs. Lillian M. Forbes (left),
Lillian E. Makle, mother (right)

BIBLIOGRAPHY

Lahita, Robert g. M.D., PhD.
Lupus Foundation of America, Inc.,
"What is Lupus?" *New York, Columbia University, 1994*

Chang-Miller, April, M.D. Mayo Clinic, Source: webpage –
https://www.mayoclinic.org, June 2011.
Buffalo Hump- Symptoms, Causes, Treatments -
https://www.healthgrades.com

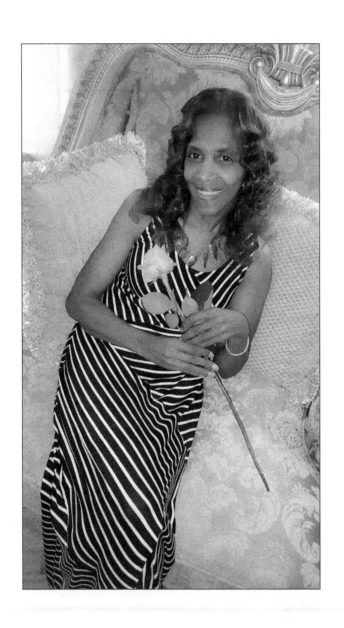

PAMPHLET SOURCES

Pamphlet: **Medical Information Series/ Systemic Lupus Erythematosus-1986**

Arthritis Foundation
1901 N. Fort Myer Drive Suite 507
Arlington, Virginia 22209

Pamphlets: **(Pamphlets and literature received from Lupus Foundation of America, 2007).**

Lupus Foundation of America Inc.
2000 L Street NW, Suite 710 Washington, DC 20036 -www.lupus.org

Types of Lupus

A. Systemic lupus erythematosus – causes inflammation in various parts of the body, most commonly the joints, kidneys, skin, brain, heart, lungs, and blood vessels. (2007)

B. Drug-induced lupus- is a lupus –like disease caused by certain prescription drugs. The drugs most commonly connected with drug-induced lupus are hydralazine (used to treat high blood pressure) procainamide (used to treat irregular heart rhythms) (2007)

C. Antiphospholipid Syndrome- leads to blood clotting disorder which leads to strokes, heart attacks and miscarriages. (2007)

D. Cutaneous lupus erythematosus – is limited to the skin, although cutaneous lupus can cause many types of rashes and lesions (sores) the most common rash is raised, scaly and red. It is called a discoid rash because because they are shaped like disks, or circles. (2007)

E. Lupus and African Americans- lupus is two to three times more prevalent among women of color, Hispanics, Asians than among Caucasian women. Recent research indicates that lupus affects 1 in 537 young African American women. (2007)

AUTHOR'S
TREATMENT LOCATIONS

Hospitals/ Dialysis Center
Georgetown University Hospital
3800 Reservoir Rd. NW, Washington, DC 20007

John Hopkins University Comprehensive Transplant Center
Kidney Pancreas Transplant Program
Post Transplant Department
720 Rutland Avenue/Turner B34
Baltimore, Maryland 21205

Fresenius Kidney Care Center
3510 Old Washington Rd Suite 300, Waldorf, Maryland 20602